The Effective Pharmacy Preceptor

Mate M. Soric, PharmD, BCPS
Clinical Pharmacy Specialist
University Hospitals Geauga Medical Center
Chardon, Ohio

Vice Chair
Practice-Based Research
Associate Professor
Pharmacy Practice
Northeast Ohio Medical University
Rootstown, Ohio

Stacey R. Schneider, PharmD
Associate Professor
Pharmacy Practice
Northeast Ohio Medical University
Rootstown, Ohio

S. Scott Wisneski, PharmD, MBA
Associate Professor
Pharmacy Practice
Northeast Ohio Medical University
Rootstown, Ohio

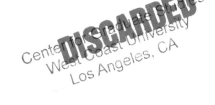
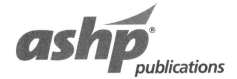

ashp publications

Any correspondence regarding this publication should be sent to the publisher, ASHP, 4500 East-West Highway, Suite 900, Bethesda, MD 20814, attention: Special Publishing.

The information presented herein reflects the opinions of the contributors and advisors. It should not be interpreted as an official policy of ASHP or as an endorsement of any product.

Because of ongoing research and improvements in technology, the information and its applications contained in this text are constantly evolving and are subject to the professional judgment and interpretation of the practitioner due to the uniqueness of a clinical situation. The editors and ASHP have made reasonable efforts to ensure the accuracy and appropriateness of the information presented in this document. However, any user of this information is advised that the editors and ASHP are not responsible for the continued currency of the information, for any errors or omissions, and/or for any consequences arising from the use of the information in the document in any and all practice settings. Any reader of this document is cautioned that ASHP makes no representation, guarantee, or warranty, express or implied, as to the accuracy and appropriateness of the information contained in this document and specifically disclaims any liability to any party for the accuracy and/or completeness of the material or for any damages arising out of the use or non-use of any of the information contained in this document.

Director, Special Publishing: Jack Bruggeman

Acquisitions Editor: Jack Bruggeman

Editorial Project Manager: Ruth Bloom

Editorial Project Manager: Bill Fogle

Cover & Page Design: Carol Barrer

Library of Congress Cataloging-in-Publication Data

Names: Soric, Mate M., author. | Schneider, Stacey R., author. | Wisneski, S. Scott, author. | American Society of Health-System Pharmacists, issuing body.
Title: The effective pharmacy preceptor / Mate M. Soric, Stacey R. Schneider,
   S. Scott Wisneski.
Description: Bethesda, MD : American Society of Health-System Pharmacists,
   [2017] | Includes bibliographical references and index.
Identifiers: LCCN 2016045570 | ISBN 9781585285549
Subjects: | MESH: Education, Pharmacy | Preceptorship | Educational Measurement
Classification: LCC RM301 | NLM QV 18 | DDC 615.1--dc23 LC record available at https://lccn.loc.gov/2016045570

ISBN: 978-1-58528-554-9

10 9 8 7 6 5 4 3 2 1

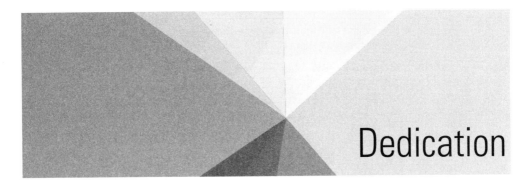

Dedication

Mate M. Soric

To my wife and family, your support throughout the writing and editing process has sustained me. To all of the preceptors from whom I learned, your example laid the foundation for the lessons contained in these pages. To my coauthors, your hard work and counsel made this book a reality.

Stacey R. Schneider

I dedicate this book to all of the preceptors and mentors who have inspired me to pursue my true passion and believed in me enough to know I would make it a reality. To all of my students who have taught me more about myself than I was able to teach them: you hold a special place in my heart. To my coauthors, I give my sincerest gratitude for providing me the opportunity to work with such brilliance, compassion, and dedication on this project.

S. Scott Wisneski

To my loving wife Diana for encouraging me through the many evenings and Sunday afternoons writing and editing this book. To all the Northeast Ohio Medical University preceptors who continually strive to provide positive learning experiences for our future pharmacists.

Table of Contents

Contributors vii

Preface ix

Part I: Building the Experience

1. The Lay of the Land: Assessing Your Practice Site for Learning Experiences 3
   Mate M. Soric

2. Tailoring the Experience 13
   S. Scott Wisneski

3. Writing Your Syllabus or Learning Experience Description 29
   Mate M. Soric

Part II: Conducting the Experience

4. Orientation 47
   Mate M. Soric

5. The Art of Teaching... 55
   Stacey R. Schneider

6. Assessing Learner Performance... 69
   S. Scott Wisneski

7. Dealing with Difficult Situations.. 87
   Stacey R. Schneider

8. Wrapping Up the Rotation 105
   S. Scott Wisneski

Part III: After the Experience

9.   Guidance Beyond the Learning Experience.. 121
     Stacey R. Schneider

10. Preceptor Assessment and Development 135
     Jaclyn Boyle

11. Using Learners to Improve Your Practice Site 147
     Lukas Everly

Index 159

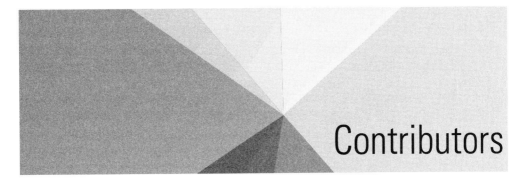

Contributors

Jaclyn Boyle, PharmD, MS, BCPS

Assistant Professor for Community
Pharmacy Innovation
Pharmacy Practice Department
Master Teacher, Master Teacher Guild
Northeast Ohio Medical University
Rootstown, Ohio

Lukas Everly, PharmD, BCPS

Assistant Clinical Professor
University of New England College of
Pharmacy
Portland, Maine

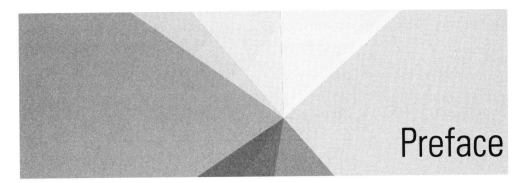

Preface

After years of preparation and training, pharmacists graduate into the healthcare environment prepared to effect meaningful improvements to patient care. We seek postgraduate training and board certification to further develop our skills. As we establish our practices and build relationships with the healthcare providers around us, we are often tasked with a challenge for which few of us are prepared: precepting pharmacists-in-training. Preceptor development is a topic rarely covered in pharmacy education, although pharmacists across the country are routinely asked to give back to their profession by precepting student and resident learners. Resources exist to help preceptors gain the skills and understand the theories of experiential education, but they are scattered across numerous sources, presented in an academic tone, or not comprehensive. As such, the quality of precepting can vary significantly from practitioner to practitioner.

In an effort to remedy this situation, we set out to create a practical, approachable guide for new and seasoned preceptors alike. *Part I, Building the Experience*, focuses on the topics of assessing a practice site for potential learning experiences, tailoring rotations to different learners, and writing a syllabus or learning experience description. *Part II, Conducting the Experience*, provides guidance for rota-

tion orientation, the best practices for delivering experiential education, learner evaluation, dealing with difficult situations, and guidance on how to effectively conclude a learning experience. *Part III, After the Experience*, goes beyond the confines of a single rotation to show where training future pharmacists fits into the big picture of your practice, with chapters covering career guidance, expansion of existing experiential offerings, and preceptor assessment.

Throughout each of the chapters you will find common elements to enhance your learning. To anchor these concepts to the real world, cases are provided that demonstrate concepts in action. *Case Questions* will be used to promote critical thinking. If you are looking at the back of the book for an answer key, look no further than the contents of the chapter you've just read, as the questions are designed to help you apply the key points to the case scenario. *Quick Tips* are also scattered throughout the text to provide precepting pearls. For the busy preceptor looking for a quick reference, flip to the back of each chapter for an element called *The Gist*. Here, the essential points of the chapter are condensed into a handful of bullet points for easy review. Finally, if you are looking for a more thorough explanation of the contents of a chapter, seek out the Suggested Reading for detailed resources.

This work would not have been possible without the hard work of our contributing authors, Jack Bruggeman, Ruth Bloom, Robin Coleman, and the rest of the incredibly hard-working ASHP publishing team. We all sincerely hope you will use what you learn here to become an effective pharmacy preceptor, shaping future generations of pharmacists to come.

Mate M. Soric
Stacey R. Schneider
S. Scott Wisneski

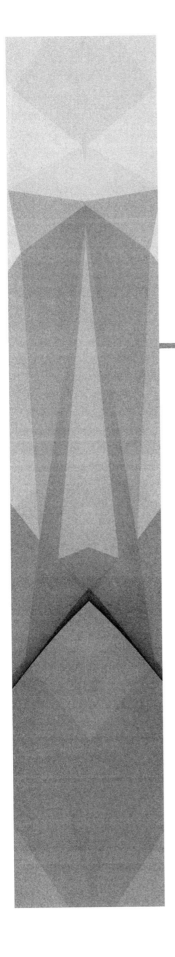

Part I

Building the Experience

1. The Lay of the Land: Assessing Your Practice Site for Learning Experiences 3
   Mate M. Soric

2. Tailoring the Experience 13
   S. Scott Wisneski

3. Writing Your Syllabus or Learning Experience Description 29
   Mate M. Soric

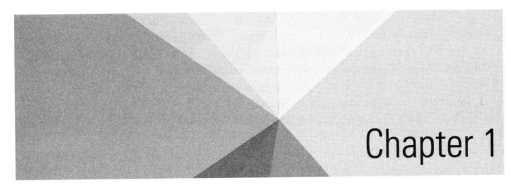

Chapter 1

The Lay of the Land: Assessing Your Practice Site for Learning Experiences

Mate M. Soric

CASE STUDY

BT is a pharmacist working in an outpatient pharmacy located in a hospital. The hospital hosts rotations for Advanced Pharmacy Practice Experience (APPE) students from a local college of pharmacy and has established a new postgraduate year 1 (PGY1) residency program. BT has been asked to establish rotations for students and residents in his unique practice setting. He is unsure of where to start and what he has to offer to these learners. He is nervous that he does not have enough activities to keep a group of learners engaged for an entire month.

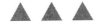

INTRODUCTION

Serving—whether choosing to serve or being chosen—as a preceptor for pharmacy students and residents can be a daunting endeavor. It can be challenging to know where to begin in the planning process, especially for new preceptors who have not developed a rotation previously. All challenges aside, however, the ability to give back to the profession in this manner provides a number of benefits to the preceptor: an avenue for keeping up to date with ever-changing medical knowledge, pharmacist extenders to help reach more patients, and a chance to give back to the profession by training the next generation of pharmacists. These benefits cannot be obtained without first deciding exactly what type of rotation you plan to host. A bit of effort and thought in advance of day one is key to a smooth learning experience that is mutually beneficial to teacher and trainee. This chapter will help you assess your practice for the kinds of activities that learners will value and compile them into an effective rotation that will go off without a hitch.

Quick Tip

The general sentiment among most new preceptors is that they feel their day-to-day job lacks exciting learning opportunities. Few realize from the start that students and residents need experience in even the mundane aspects of pharmacy practice and will find value in your guidance.

ASSESSING THE STRENGTHS OF YOUR PRACTICE

When thinking of activities and opportunities for future students, the best place to begin tends to be your site's strengths. The things you do particularly well are the low-hanging fruit for experiential rotations. They will require little effort on your part to model exemplary behavior, and you are likely already an expert in the development, day-to-day operations, and assessment of these services. The only missing piece is the learner to soak up the knowledge you have to offer.

Consider the services your site is particularly proud of, such as:

◆ Pharmacist-provided patient care services
◆ Medical teams that have good relationships or regular interactions with pharmacists
◆ Committees that feature prominent pharmacy involvement
◆ Advanced technologies that your department utilizes that students may not have had exposure to in their didactic curriculum

By identifying these strengths, you can begin to get a sense of the framework on which to build your rotation.

While brainstorming the foundational activities for your rotation, remember that you can look beyond the walls of your institution for extra activities that could be of significant value to your students. Do you deliver lectures at a local college of pharmacy? Consider bringing learners into your lecture planning, developing exam items, and classroom delivery. The change of pace can be refreshing for students who have not had experience on the other side of the lectern. Supplementary preceptors may also be identified from within the pharmacy department or from other professions that can offer alternative viewpoints to the student or resident. Although a pharmacist should be the primary preceptor for students and residents, consider enlisting the help of technicians, nurses, physicians, surgeons, dietitians, social workers, or physical therapists to give your trainees a well-rounded view of patient care in your setting. For examples of the potential roles of supplemental preceptors, see Table 1-1.

Quick Tip

When using nonpharmacist preceptors for pharmacy residents, you must document that the resident can perform the duties of a pharmacist in the patient care area independently before the start of a rotation. In addition to these requirements, the nonpharmacist and a pharmacist must collaboratively develop the learning experience to ensure the preceptor understands the expectations of a pharmacist in that setting.

ASSESSING THE WEAKNESSES OF YOUR PRACTICE

If you simply dwell on the strengths of your site, although easier to do than considering the weaknesses, you will leave considerable gaps in your planning process. You should also assess the weaknesses of your practice site to anticipate future problems and avoid them, if possible. First, consider logistical issues that could arise. In general, most pharmacy departments do not have ample space available to house learners. For residents,

Table 1-1. Sample Supplemental Preceptor-Led Learning Activities

Supplemental Preceptor	Potential Learning Activities
Pharmacy technician	Fill, maintain, and prepare audits of robotic prescription dispensing systems
Patient safety officer	Complete Failure Mode and Effects Analyses or practice patient tracers
Cardiologist	Observe cardiac catheterizations
Social worker	Observe and complete patient assistance program applications
Dietitian	Participate in total parenteral nutrition assessments and adjustments
Skilled nursing facility nurse	Participate in new patient assessments and medication reviews
Laboratory manager	Review the processing and interpretation of microbiological culture and sensitivity
Physical therapist	Identify nonpharmacological treatment options for musculoskeletal issues

dedicated office space is a must, but for students, creative solutions might be needed to provide work space. With regard to technology, it is helpful to plan exactly how learners will gain access to computer systems, electronic medical records, and drug information resources in advance of the rotation's start date. Levels of access can sometimes hamper your student's ability to access all information needed to provide patient care or document their activities. With regard to patient care activities, consider potential issues with patient load (whether there are too many patients or too few), availability of additional preceptors to provide backup to primary preceptors who may be pulled away from rotation activities, and issues occurring between departments that could negatively affect learning. Anticipating these potential issues before learners arrive on site can help you avoid difficult or embarrassing situations and will lead to a smoother rotation.

The weaknesses of your practice should not always be seen as threats. Weaknesses can also serve as opportunities for growth in your department and as a source of projects for learners. When you feel you are falling short of providing the required care, your trainees can be assigned to evaluate best practices, scour the literature for solutions, and develop pilot programs to help move your services to the next level. When implementing new services, students and residents can act as trainers for existing staff, lessening the burden on the pharmacists that would otherwise be responsible for getting the staff on board. Residents, in particular, are required by accreditation standards to complete a project over the course of the year. By identifying the practice site's weaknesses, you have likely also developed a list of potential projects for your learners. The net result is mutually beneficial to the trainee, the practice site, and may even be disseminated to other practices via poster presentations and manuscripts (thus improving the practice of pharmacy as a whole).

Case Question

BT has been working hard to establish new medication therapy management (MTM) services in his outpatient pharmacy. The results have been impressive, and he feels the service is making a real impact. His other duties in the pharmacy include filling prescriptions and serving as the vice chair of the pharmacy and therapeutics committee. BT really wishes that his pharmacy could offer a bedside delivery service for inpatients, but does not have the resources to implement the service at this time. How could a trainee benefit from this site's strengths, weaknesses, and day-to-day activities?

USING GOALS AND OBJECTIVES AS A FRAMEWORK

Thus far, the activities you have identified as potentially beneficial to trainees are a loosely connected group of tasks without much organization. Connecting these activities into a framework allows your rotation to become more structured and will help you identify areas of the rotation that require some extra development. When developing a rotation, you will likely receive some considerable help from the experiential director at the colleges or schools of pharmacy sending students and from the ASHP Accreditation Standards for pharmacy residents. These resources will provide you with a list of goals and objectives that are essentially a description of the knowledge, skills, and attitudes that they expect their learners to develop while on rotation. Knowing these expectations up front will allow you to develop your rotation with the end goal in mind. Working backward from these goals and objectives, you can begin to connect the loose list of activities identified above to the anticipated outcomes of your training, leading to a cohesive, thoughtful approach to rotation development.

Many preceptors find it beneficial to create a grid containing all assigned goals and objectives listed vertically in a column. In the adjacent columns, create a list of the specific activities that will be used to teach and assess your student or resident's progress toward the assigned goals and objectives (see Table 1-2). Be diligent in specifically listing activities. Avoid broad terms such as *patient care* or *dispensing* in favor of the specific tasks that would exemplify the proper knowledge or skills required of a pharmacist. It is also important to evaluate the verbs used in the goals and objectives. Most often, Bloom's *Taxonomy*[1] (or another taxonomy) is utilized to identify cognitive levels (or the level of proficiency) for each objective.[2] Objectives can be written with an eye toward the learner gaining foundational knowledge, applying his or her knowledge, creating something new, or practicing independently. Use caution to pair activities at the appropriate level for the objective at hand. For instance, assigning a reading activity to an objective that states students must accurately identify all medication-related problems is a mismatch. Instead, the preceptor should provide an opportunity for the learner to work up a patient case and create a problem list. Discussions and readings are appropriate activities for recall or knowledge-based objectives but would be inappropriate for application-based objectives.

Case Question

BT is creating a grid to connect his learning activities to the goals and objective of his rotation. What type of rotation activity would best fit with the learning objective: "Create a monitoring plan to assess the outcomes of drug therapy for a patient?" Would a discussion with the preceptor on the concept be adequate to teach and assess this objective?

Once the document contains all of your planned activities, a quick scan across all of the columns can help you identify any goals or objectives that are poorly linked to the planned activities (or contain no linked activity at all). Identifying these gaps early on in the planning process is key to avoiding an underperforming rotation. Completing this exercise before trainees are on site will help you identify gaps and put a plan together to fill them before learners arrive. Filling gaps may not always be an easy process and may require a degree of creativity from the preceptors involved in the rotation. Consider looking to additional preceptors, extra projects, assigned readings or developing new services to fill these gaps, always remembering to consider the level of the verb in the objective. If you are unable to identify any activities to fill the gaps, you may be able to request a change to the assigned goals and objectives. Seek out the advice of the experiential director or the residency program director for more help.

Table 1-2. Sample Learning Objective Grid

Learning Objectives	Learning Activities		
Interact effectively with patients, family members, and caregivers	Conduct MTM visits with new and established patients	Provide counseling to patients, families, and caregivers picking up new and refilled prescriptions	
Collect information on which to base safe and effective medication therapy	Complete a thorough patient interview during each MTM visit	Complete a chart review before each MTM visit to gather pertinent data	Review refill history for each MTM patient before their visit to assess adherence
Design or redesign safe and effective patient-centered therapeutic regimens and monitoring plans (care plans)	Create a therapeutic plan based on appropriate guidelines and patient-specific data (with drug, dose, route, frequency, and duration)	Choose appropriate monitoring parameters for safety and efficacy endpoints	During follow-up visits, review all interventions for continued efficacy and safety
Document direct patient care activities appropriately in the medical record or where appropriate	Discuss proper documentation techniques with the preceptor	Review preceptor's documentation technique after each MTM visit	
Prepare and dispense medications following best practices and the organization's policies and procedures	Safely prepare compounded medications, such as suspensions, creams, and oral vancomycin	Use the prospective drug use review system to assess orders for appropriateness and safety	
Manage aspects of the medication-use process related to oversight of dispensing	Provide the final verification for technicians' completed orders		
Develop a plan to improve the patient care and/ or the medication-use system	Create a business plan for a bedside delivery program		

In the course of your planning process, you may also come across activities that do not fit with any of the assigned objectives. This may not always be a bad thing. First, examine the number of unmatched activities. If there are a large number of them, perhaps the rotation you are planning to offer does not match the expectation of the college of pharmacy or your residency program director. Ensure that the rotation has been classified correctly; a clinical rotation will have a very different set of expectations when compared to a leadership rotation. Next, examine the utility of each unmatched activity closely. If there is significant benefit offered to the learners that complete these activities, it may be perfectly reasonable to include the activity in the rotation. For residents, you may even create your own objective to allow for assessment of these skills. Accreditation standards allow for the creation of elective objectives so that residency programs can tailor their assessment strategy to unique offerings at each practice site. Keep in mind, however, that all of the same rules apply to both elective and required objectives (with regard to learning taxonomy, assessment, and measurability). Any activity that does not contribute substantially to the learner's development is truly extraneous and should be removed from the rotation. By the end of this planning activity, a complete list of rotation activities will be created that meets the needs of your learners, highlights the strengths of your practice, and accounts for potential issues that may arise.

Case Question

BT has created a grid of his future resident's required goals and objectives and has linked the activities he has planned for the rotation (see Table 1-2). What gaps can you identify that will require attention?

DEVELOPING DAY-TO-DAY ACTIVITIES

Once you have a finalized list of activities, you can begin to arrange them into a tentative schedule for the rotation. When establishing the schedule for a typical rotation day, consider what times of day contain the bulk of your activities. Depending on your setting, a typical 9:00 a.m. to 5:00 p.m. day may not be optimal for learning. In most cases, you are also not confined to business hours. If the action occurs during off-hours or weekends, it may be best to adjust the start and end times of the rotation accordingly. Arrange your planned activities into a calendar or day planner to allow for visualization of the learner's workday. Time should also be set aside for topic discussions and learner assessments at regular intervals during the experience. Ensure your list of activities is not overly ambitious and can easily be accomplished in the time allotted to your rotation. If the activities exceed the hours in the day, some prioritization of activities or simplification of the rotation can go a long way toward keeping your learners happy and engaged.

Quick Tip

When creating the day-to-day schedule for your rotations, consider including some free time to allow for project or presentation work to occur onsite. Giving your learners this opportunity to work on larger assignments on site allows them to reach out to you directly in the event there are miscommunications or misunderstanding about the expectations.

As you build the learner's schedule, it is also important to simultaneously identify the opportunities for preceptor interaction. The amount of preceptor oversight will vary dramatically depending on the learner's level and skill set; however, it is very helpful to establish a baseline plan for preceptor involvement that can be adjusted once the trainees arrive. By preplanning your involvement, you will have a better idea if the tentative schedule allows for adequate teaching opportunities or whether adjustments are necessary. Similarly, you will have the chance to identify if the planned activities require too much preceptor oversight that might become a burden over time and lead to preceptor burnout and poor performance during the rotation.

One last bit of preplanning to consider is a curriculum of topics to address over the course of the rotation. This helps to ensure that important topics are not overlooked and standardizes the rotation from trainee to trainee. Topics can be addressed in the course of the activities you have assigned, in reading assignments or in dedicated topic discussions led by the preceptor or the trainees. Although direct instruction is generally minimized during rotations in favor of modeling, coaching, and facilitation, discussions can be useful for catching topics that may have been missed due to the natural ebb and flow of activities or disease states over the course of a year. (For more information on the preceptor roles of direct instruction, modeling, coaching, and facilitation, see Chapter 5.)

CONTINGENCY PROJECTS

Having a schedule is an important part of the planning process, but life happens. When unforeseen issues arise in the course of a rotation, it is very helpful to have a list of contingency projects available to be assigned to learners in the case of unexpected delays, downtime, or disasters. The types of projects included on the list can be extensive and vary by the type of rotation you are offering. Options to consider include:

- Additional readings
- Drug information papers
- Quizzes or exams
- Working on inventory issues
- Creating or maintaining a bank of recorded lectures for learners to access and view, when needed

It may also be acceptable to grant additional work time if a number of projects have already been assigned. In this manner, you can be prepared with an ace up your sleeve whenever the unexpected strikes.

ASSESSING YOUR OWN STRENGTHS AND WEAKNESSES

Thus far, the planning process for a new rotation has centered largely on evaluating your practice site, identifying activities, and building tentative schedules. The final step in the planning process requires an evaluation of the preceptor who will be hosting the experience. Although it may not always be the most enjoyable activity, self-reflection and assessment are vital to hosting a good rotation.

Some questions to consider when evaluating your readiness for taking learners include:

♦ What are your inherent biases and how might they affect your trainees?
♦ Why did you choose to precept learners?
♦ What do you do particularly well that should be passed on to your learners?
♦ What are your own knowledge gaps and how do you plan on addressing them?
♦ How will you handle difficult conversations with your trainees?

Completing an honest self-evaluation is key to anticipating potential issues and will further prepare you for a smooth rotation and satisfied learners.

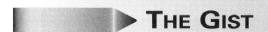 **THE GIST**

1. Objectively assess your practice site for strengths and weaknesses.
   a. The strengths are an excellent initial list of rotation activities for learners.
   b. Weaknesses should be considered to identify issues before they arise; some can become projects for learners to work on improving.
2. Use college/school of pharmacy and residency goals and objectives to identify your rotation's expectations.
3. Working backward, link each goal/objective to an activity you plan to use to teach and evaluate those skills.
4. From this list of activities, plan out a typical day to ensure enough time will be available to complete all identified activities.
5. Have contingency projects lined up in case of unexpected delays, downtime, or possible disasters.

SUGGESTED READING

Kelley KW, McBane, S, Thomas T et al. Serving as a preceptor to pharmacy students: Tips on maintaining the desire to inspire. *Am J Health Syst Pharm.* 2012; 69:826-31.

Lagasse C, Wilkinson S, Buck B et al. Integrating precepting into your daily practice. *Hosp Pharm.* 2013; 48(3):200-3.

REFERENCES

1. Bloom BS. *Taxonomy of Educational Objectives Book 1: Cognitive Domain.* 2nd ed. White Plains, NY: Longman; 1984.
2. Krathwohl DR, Bloom BS, Masia BB. *Taxonomy of Educational Objectives, The Classification of Educational Goals, Handbook II: Affective Domain.* New York: David McKay; 1956.

Chapter 2

Tailoring the Experience

S. Scott Wisneski

CASE STUDY

SK is an acute care clinical pharmacist at a 300-bed community teaching hospital. She currently serves as a preceptor for a postgraduate year 1 (PGY1) pharmacy practice resident and periodically will take advanced pharmacy practice experience (APPE) students from the local college of pharmacy for 2-month experiences. Recently, the pharmacy management team decided to expand the number of student rotation offerings to include introductory pharmacy practice experiences (IPPEs). The intent of this initiative is to utilize students to assist in the department's newly created transitions of care program. SK is concerned that the increased number of students she precepts will jeopardize her ability to provide an effective experience for the resident and the students. She is also unfamiliar with the requirements for students completing IPPEs.

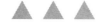

INTRODUCTION

As health systems create new or enhance existing patient care services, pharmacies are exploring the role students can have in these initiatives. In the era of decreasing staffing levels, students can help in the delivery of advanced services. As a result, a preceptor may be responsible for training a greater number of students who are often at different stages in their education. The variability in acquired knowledge, practice-related skill experience, and level of professionalism in pharmacy students and residents can be challenging for a preceptor to provide effective learning experiences. You must consider the needs of individual students and, thus, provide different experiences to help students and residents grow in their development. Managing students and residents simultaneously is a tremendous responsibility often fraught with increased workload and frustration for the preceptor, who feels the strain of precepting while trying to accomplish day-to-day activities, such as patient care. Strategies such as the layered learning model (LLM) can be an effective way for today's preceptor to manage students and residents at the same time.

INTRODUCTORY PHARMACY PRACTICE EXPERIENCES

Encompassing no less than 300 hr (5% of the doctor of pharmacy curriculum), IPPEs expose students to common practice models, including interprofessional practice involving shared patient care decision making, professional ethics, expected behaviors, and direct patient care activities.[1] At least 50% of the IPPE hours should be balanced between community and institutional practice settings. Occurring early and continuing throughout the student's didactic training, IPPEs are designed to facilitate knowledge application and clinical reasoning skills, as well as prepare students for the APPEs completed at the end of their training.[2] Colleges and schools of pharmacy will vary in the structure, schedule, and type of experiences the students will complete in their respective IPPE programs. Although the majority of IPPEs often focus on operational aspects of practice, such as dispensing and compounding medications, some may include community service, preventative health screenings, health fairs, and simulations. Through exposure to pharmacy practitioners and support personnel, IPPEs are also essential for the students' professional socialization, allowing them to see and exhibit professional behavior essential for today's practice.

Students completing IPPEs possess different characteristics than more advanced students. Some IPPE students may present with only an introductory knowledge of common medications, disease states, pharmacology, and therapeutics; some have had no practice experience prior to starting an IPPE, while others may have worked in a pharmacy prior to starting their education. Students on these rotations will likely have experiences limited to one practice setting, if they have any experience at all. Given the limited knowledge and experience, the IPPE rotation must be designed to progressively develop the students' competence in essential skills. Schools of pharmacy can provide their preceptors with specific goals and objectives for the IPPEs, which are often based on the students' current and expected levels of development. With this information, you can determine the appropriate activities the students will perform while at your practice site. Table 2-1 provides suggested activities often performed during institution- and community-based IPPEs. Note this list is not all inclusive, and the preceptor should consider including additional activities he or she believes would benefit the students.

Table 2-1. Patient Care Activities for IPPEs
Institution-Based IPPEs
Participate in the medication distribution process to include evaluation of the process for improvement
Prepare sterile products using aseptic technique and performing required calculations
Describe the role and responsibilities of the personnel in the pharmacy
Perform patient medication reconciliation
Observe and participate in discharge counseling of patients
Attend patient care rounds with a clinical pharmacist or resident
Identify the common medications used in institutional practice
Community-Based IPPEs
Participate in the processing and dispensing of new and refill prescriptions
Compound nonsterile medications and perform required calculations
Collect patient medical histories
Observe and perform patient medication counseling and disease state education
Participate in patient care services, including pharmacy-run immunization services and MTM
Participate in the billing of third-party insurance programs
Institution- and Community-Based IPPEs
Respond to drug information inquiries
Identify and report adverse drug reactions
Detect medication errors
Protect patient health-related information
Participate in discussion of a journal club
Participate in pharmacy department meetings
Write an article for a pharmacy newsletter

Generally, students starting IPPEs will have little awareness of the different types of practice settings employing pharmacists. In addition, the vast majority will not have made any formal decisions about the type of practice they will pursue on graduation. The IPPEs are an ideal opportunity for students to be exposed to different practice settings. You should introduce and explain how your practice compares and contrasts with other settings. Consider discussing why you pursued your particular practice. This can include discussion around the future opportunities and potential threats to the practice. Students find this information extremely helpful as they start to consider the type of practice they will seek as they finish their schooling.

In addition to gaining knowledge and developing practice experience during an IPPE, students will also be able to further refine their own professional behavior. The students may only have had some lectures on the subject and not yet had the opportunity to exhibit professionalism in a real-life pharmacy practice setting. At this stage in their training, the students may be naive to the expectations or consequences of exhibiting unprofessional behavior. The preceptor plays an important role in assessing and guiding the students' professionalism. Anticipate that there will be situations ranging from being tardy to more serious infractions, such as a breach of patient confidentiality, in which students will exhibit a behavior that is less than desirable for practice. Guide your students by providing clear expectations for professionalism, including the potential ramifications for behavior deemed unacceptable. Consider covering the importance of proper dress, grooming, timeliness, and use of cellular devices on day one of your rotation. Empathy, altruism, cultural competence, sense of duty, and lifelong learning are also important traits to discuss and assess in your students. Because students are quite impressionable at this stage, you need to be cognizant of your own behavior as well. Being a positive role model will help to ensure the students are developing into the type of pharmacists for which our profession is known.

Quick Tip

Have your students describe key characteristics of being a professional, including empathy, altruism, cultural competence, sense of duty, responsibility, and lifelong learning. Discuss how your own description compares and contrasts to what the students provided.

The IPPEs are an opportunity for students to develop their skills in counseling patients and interacting with healthcare professionals. Their colleges of pharmacy may have provided simulations to help develop and assess communication skills. However, simulation cannot replace the real-life encounters. Students may initially find counseling patients or talking to physicians uncomfortable and challenging, resulting in timid interactions and a lack of confidence. The preceptor plays an important role in coaching and providing opportunities for students to develop good communication skills. Early on, the students should observe your interactions with patients and providers. You should discuss these encounters with the students, providing suggestions on proper techniques in effective communication. The students should then be given the opportunity to demonstrate these skills while being closely monitored. Allow time for constructive feedback, indicating what went well and what improvements are needed in future encounters.

Students completing an IPPE may exhibit skills associated with dependent learners. With limited training and experience, the students tend to rely heavily on the preceptor to instruct and guide them through each activity. Students may not be fully aware of the gaps in their knowledge and, as a result, lack confidence to perform certain activities independently. An effective preceptor can initially explain how a particular task is done, demonstrate the task, watch the students perform the task, and then allow the students to perform the task independently. The sink or swim method of learning is not recommended at this stage, especially the first time the student is completing an activity. Continually assessing the progression of your students will help you to keep them engaged and give the opportunity to assign new activities. If students are performing at a high level, allow for more challenging activities. Feedback will help students continue to build their skills and progress to the next level. Over time, more confidence will develop, and the students will become more independent learners.

Preparing to host an IPPE, a preceptor needs to:

- Review the structure, schedule, and objectives of the IPPE from the school of pharmacy
- Identify a variety of activities the students can complete to meet each objective for the IPPE
- Prepare a list of professionalism-related expectations
- Develop an orientation for the first day the students arrive
- Create a plan for assessment and provision of feedback for the students

Preceptors should provide a warm welcome, using orientation to help relieve any anxiety the students may be experiencing as well as set the tone for the rotation. Consider that this may be the first time your student is exposed to your practice setting. An effective orientation should provide an overview of the practice setting, tour of the pharmacy, and introductions to the pharmacy staff. Additionally, a schedule of activities, required assignments, expectations for performance, and the assessment process should be provided (refer to Chapter 3 for more information). The orientation is an opportunity to ask the students about their past work or training in a pharmacy, their professional interests, and their own goals for the experience. The preceptor should attempt to provide activities that meet the IPPE objectives while considering the students' previous experience and interests.

Although assessment is an important part of any rotation, IPPEs, in particular, need additional guidance and oversight. Being available to answer questions and provide additional instruction, when needed, will go a long way in meeting learning needs. It is essential that the preceptor provide students consistent and on-going feedback during the rotation. Students want to know if their performance is meeting the expectations of the preceptor and where improvement is needed. Chapter 6 provides a more in-depth look at delivering effective feedback to students.

Case Question

SK's typical day consists of morning patient care rounds with the internal medicine team along with the PGY1 resident and any APPE students present. The afternoon is devoted to following up on patient-related issues, conducting topic discussions with the resident and students, attending meetings, and working on projects. She also assists in the main pharmacy a few afternoons each week processing medication orders. Starting next month, she will have a second-year pharmacy student scheduled to complete a 64-hr IPPE, 1 day per week for 8 weeks. The college of pharmacy has provided her a list of objectives focused on general pharmacy operations, drug information, and counseling patients. What types of activities can the second-year student perform that will benefit his learning at SK's practice site?

ADVANCED PHARMACY PRACTICE EXPERIENCES

APPEs are designed to integrate, apply, reinforce, and advance the knowledge, skills, attitudes, abilities, and behaviors developed in the pre-APPE curriculum.[1] APPEs total no less than 36 weeks or 1,440 hr of practice experiences completed during the student's final year of the degree program.

Required APPEs occur in four practice settings:

1. Community pharmacy
2. Ambulatory patient care
3. Hospital/health-system pharmacy
4. Inpatient general medicine patient care

Remaining APPEs will include elective experiences focused on clinical pharmacy specialties (e.g., cardiology, infectious disease, psychiatry, pediatrics), practice management, research, drug information, compounding, pharmaceutical industry, professional association management, and various others.

Depending on the college of pharmacy's program, APPEs are generally completed in 4- to 8-week blocks at approximately 40 hr per week. Students starting their APPEs have completed their formal didactic training with at least 300 hr of IPPEs, and most will have gained additional experience as interns in a community or hospital setting. At this point, the students should have some familiarity with different practice settings and developed basic competency in dispensing and the medication-use process of your type practice setting. In addition, the students will have had the opportunity to counsel patients, interact with prescribers, and may have participated in patient-centered care activities such as administration of immunizations, medication therapy management, and therapeutic care plan development. APPEs are intended to place a greater emphasis on patient-centered care activities, exposure to diverse patient populations, and delivery of care as part of an interprofessional team. Some IPPE-related activities may occur during APPEs, but the majority of the time should be focused on patient-centered skills. Table 2-2 lists suggested patient-centered care activities often performed during an APPE.

Additional activities that are commonly completed during APPEs include:

- Journal club presentations
- Patient case presentations
- Topic discussions
- Preparation of a new drug monograph
- Management-related activities
- Research or writing projects

Students starting an APPE will generally have little experience working up complex patient care cases or completing in-depth problem solving. It is imperative for the effective preceptor to create an advanced experience that helps to foster critical thinking. Your focus should provide evidence-based, patient-centered rationale for drug therapy recommendations. This can be accomplished through student-led patient cases and disease state topic discussions. The preceptor should ask thought-provoking questions during these activities to assess and further develop the students' thinking skills.

Prior to the APPEs, the students have largely been dependent learners. This is an ideal time for the preceptor to encourage and reinforce independent learning. The students should develop confidence interacting directly with patients and prescribers.

Table 2-2. Patient-Centered Care Activities for Community- and Institution-Based APPEs

Community-Based APPEs

Participate in patient counseling and education

Provide patient care-related services (e.g., MTM, antibiotic call-back program, chronic medication refill reminders, administer immunizations)

Perform physical assessments (e.g., blood pressure screening, blood glucose/cholesterol checks)

Assess medication adherence

Answer drug information questions

Prepare community education presentations (e.g., brown bag event, poison prevention, medication-related topic)

Develop new patient care or value-added service

Institution-Based APPEs

Perform medication reconciliation

Provide patient discharge medication counseling

Perform patient assessments

Answer drug information questions

Participate in patient care interprofessional team rounds

Assess drug therapy and making recommendations to prescribers

Although the preceptor should anticipate most students will lack confidence and assertiveness (especially early on in these type of interactions), providing the students with the opportunity to counsel patients, make recommendations to physicians, and interact with a medical team are ideal ways to foster their confidence and help them develop independence.

Quick Tip

Have your students present a short presentation to the medical team on a drug-related problem identified during rounds. Encourage team members to ask questions related to the presentation. Follow up by asking the students to provide their impressions and self-assessment of the activity.

The APPEs are an opportunity for students to further develop their professionalism. Transitioning from primarily didactic to full-time experiential training may be difficult for some students. They need to prioritize and manage their time appropriately to accomplish the rotation's tasks. It is easy to fall behind in completing assignments on time. The preceptor must set clear expectations and deadlines as well as provide suggestions on how best to manage time. Students must develop a process for self-assessment and display an interest in continuous professional development. Have them reflect on their performance and identify areas that need improvement to help your students develop this skill. Reinforce with the students the duty to review any didactic knowledge that may have been lost or never learned. You should not be expected to teach your students information that has been previously taught in the classroom. Challenge your students to research a drug- or disease state–related question that likely was not covered in the curriculum to get them accustomed to continuous learning. Remember to also assess other areas of professionalism, including empathy toward patients, professional appearance, patient confidentiality, and cultural sensitivity.

Aspects to consider in preparation for an APPE are similar to those for an IPPE. You should review the goals and objectives of the experience provided by the college or school of pharmacy. Key activities should be planned to meet and assess each objective. Because the students will be at the practice site full-time for at least a month, a calendar of activities, assignments, presentations, and evaluations should be drafted and shared with the pharmacy staff. Consider allowing the students' input into the types of activities to include on the calendar (within reason). This allows for alternative or additional activities that the students would like to accomplish during the rotation. Preceptors are encouraged to prepare a written syllabus for the APPE. See Chapter 3 for additional information about creating your syllabus.

Be sure to schedule time to learn about your students' professional backgrounds, experiences, and interests. You should request the students' curriculum vitae, portfolios (if available), and prior rotation evaluations. The objective is to have an appreciation of the students' strengths and weaknesses so you can provide an effective experience. Finally, there should be a plan for assessing and evaluating students. The school of pharmacy will have evaluation forms (often completed on line) for you to use. Review the specific items on the evaluation before your students start the rotation. Midpoint and final evaluations should be scheduled and communicated to the students.

Case Question

SK's APPE student has completed only an advanced community rotation and a long-term care elective prior to starting this internal medicine experience. The student expresses a desire to gain more experience evaluating drug therapy and making recommendations to physicians. What types of activities can SK have her student complete to gain the experience? How would SK assess this skill over the course of the rotation?

POSTGRADUATE YEAR 1 RESIDENCY

According the ASHP 2014 accreditation standards, a PGY1 residency program builds on the doctor of pharmacy (PharmD) education and outcomes to contribute to the development of clinical pharmacists responsible for medication-related care of patients with a wide range of conditions, eligible for board certification, and eligible for postgraduate year 2 (PGY2) pharmacy residency training.[3] PGY1 residents acquire knowledge for effective problem solving, strengthen their professional values and attitudes, and advance their clinical judgment.

On completion of the program, the PGY1 resident should demonstrate competency in the following four areas:

1. Patient care
2. Advancing practice and improving patient care
3. Leadership and management
4. Teaching, education, and dissemination of knowledge

At the start of the residency program, a baseline assessment of the residents should be conducted. A survey and/or discussion with the residents can ideally gather information on their prior experiences, strengths, accomplishments, and areas of needed development. In addition, assessment tools such as VARK Questionnaire, Kolb Learning Style Inventory, the Health Professionals' Inventory, or Learning Styles (H-PILS) may provide further information for the assessment.[4-6] From the baseline assessment, you can create a developmental plan for your residents. The plan should also include their personal goals for the year, career goals, and professional interests. Preceptors can use this plan to expose the residents to activities that improve weaknesses, enhance strengths, and align with goals and career interests.

The PGY1 residents' characteristics are different than those of pharmacy students completing an APPE. For the first time, the individual is assuming the accountability that comes with being a licensed pharmacist. This must be balanced with the plethora of activities that will be accomplished during a residency. Residents are typically eager to learn, desire to get the most out of their residency program, and are often unwilling to say "no" when new opportunities are presented. It is common for the residents to strive for perfection and, as a result, may spend excessive time on or procrastinate in completing assignments. Time and opportunity management can serve as the greatest need of improvement for the PGY1 residents. The preceptor can help the residents focus their time based on the particular task's importance and urgency. For example, an activity of high importance and urgency should be prioritized above lower-level tasks.

Quick Tip

Determine the time and opportunity management considerations you can incorporate into your rotations. Think about the rotation's structure, the activities assigned to the resident, the resident's responsibilities to the site, and the resident's development plan. Identifying time management challenges ahead of time will help you guide your resident through the process of developing these skills more effectively.

PGY1 residents provide the practice site with the potential opportunity to expand patient care services, complete quality improvement projects, increase research initiatives, and provide additional coverage of operations. The preceptor needs to be careful to assign tasks that align with the site's priorities and the residents' own interests and development. The preceptor should ensure the residents are involved in all activities in which a pharmacist can partake, including precepting students. At the beginning of the residency, the preceptor may want to set specific expectations regarding time spent at the site and assignment deadlines. As the year progresses, the preceptor may want to lessen these requirements for the residents and focus more on performance boundaries. In the end, this will help foster the residents' autonomy. As the residents' learning progresses, the preceptor's role should also evolve from direct instruction and modeling to more coaching and facilitating. See Chapter 5 for more discussion on preceptor roles.

Quick Tip

PGY1 residents will also need to develop an ability to anticipate the next steps for a given situation. The ability to think two steps ahead is an advanced skill that will be invaluable to the residents as they establish their practice. Try having your residents predict the next likely scenario or issue that may occur. Examples of this include the anticipated response to a new medication administered to a patient, likely questions from the audience of a formal presentation, how a physician may react to a medication recommendation, or how the staff pharmacists will react to a new patient care service. The abilities to anticipate reactions, outcomes, and next steps are essential skills the residents need to develop.

The residents may also struggle with knowing when a task has been completed. Although the residents' completion of some activities may be apparent and finite (e.g., conducting a point-of-care test, administering an immunization, or determining the renal dose of a drug), the completion of others may be harder to determine. The residents may spend what appear to be endless hours researching a drug information question not realizing the need for a more timely response. In some situations, this could delay needed patient care. This type of behavior is common in those who are perfectionists by nature. The preceptor must provide coaching to break the tendency of residents becoming paralyzed by the thought of any error or shortcoming of a task leading to needless delay.

It may be the preceptor's desire for the PGY1 residents to develop expertise in a particular therapeutic area. Remember that these residencies are intended to develop core competence in a broad range of essential clinical skills rather than expertise in a specific area. PGY1 residencies build on the knowledge, skills, attitudes, and abilities that were obtained in the PharmD curriculum. You should help your resident build competency in medication-use systems and an ability to optimize drug therapy outcomes in patients with a variety of disorders. Further specialization is the purpose of a PGY2 residency year.

In a nutshell, the preceptor needs to have their residents concentrate on the personal and professional development that aligns with their career goals. Celebrate the successes in performance, especially when overcoming a challenge. Develop and improve the residents' shortcomings while encouraging them to try again when something does not go as expected.

POSTGRADUATE YEAR 2 RESIDENCY

PGY2 residency training is a program which builds on the PharmD education and PGY1 residency programs to contribute to the development of clinical pharmacists in specialized areas of practice (e.g., pediatrics, infectious disease, critical care, cardiology, psychiatry, ambulatory care, oncology). ASHP provides program outcomes and educational objectives for different PGY2 residencies.[7] These residencies provide the opportunity to function independently as practitioners by conceptualizing knowledge and integrating accumulated experience and knowledge and incorporating both into the provision of patient care that improves medication therapy.[8] Residents who successfully complete a PGY2 residency should possess competencies that qualify them for a clinical pharmacist and/or faculty position and be in a position to obtain a board certification in a specialized practice area (if it exists).[8]

A key objective of a PGY2 residency program is for residents to demonstrate the ability to function independently as clinical pharmacists. To accomplish this goal, the preceptor has to allow the residents to function with a relatively higher level of autonomy compared to students and PGY1 residents, although a balanced level of oversight from the preceptor needs to remain to ensure quality patient care is maintained. Initially, the preceptor will place some limits on the residents but, as soon as they demonstrate an acceptable level of skill, the autonomy should increase.

The ability to work independently can be developed through key activities occurring in practice. The PGY2 residents should take the lead with educational sessions or topic discussions for other students. The residents may choose the topic, provide resources to students, and lead the discussion. Not only does this foster autonomy, but it also provides the residents with an opportunity to demonstrate competency in teaching others. The preceptor should avoid the tendency to control the discussion but provide input, correct mistakes, and compliment high-quality work.

The residents' autonomy should be most evident in the delivery of patient care. They should be able to manage a full patient load as well as be an active participant on the medical team. As more students and PGY1 residents become involved with patient care activities, the PGY2 residents should take an active role in precepting these less-experienced learners, which will develop the residents' teaching and leadership skills. It also helps to free up time for the preceptor to focus on other responsibilities.

A PGY2 resident's independence can be further enhanced through completion of quality improvement and research projects. As a requirement of any residency program, residents should design and implement quality improvement changes with a class of drugs, medication-use evaluation, or medication safety concern. Through this activity, the residents gain experience and competence in assisting an institution to make quality improvements. Compared to a PGY1's project, a PGY2 resident's research project should include developing the research idea and protocol preparation and establishing all deadlines. The preceptor's role is to allow the residents to work more autonomously while also providing coaching. A preceptor should intervene only when a particular project is not going as planned. By taking this approach, the preceptor helps to facilitate the residents' ability to function as independent clinical pharmacists.

LAYERED LEARNING MODEL

As pharmacies face the challenge of decreasing revenues, increased accountability for patient outcomes, and the pressure of doing more with less, the use of student pharmacists and residents to assist in providing patient care services is becoming more prevalent. In 2013, ASHP approved a policy that supports pharmacy practice training models that use students in teams and recognizes student pharmacists in providing direct patient care when overseen by a supervising pharmacist.[9] Students and residents can offer significant benefits to health systems by providing patient care services such as medication reconciliation, direct patient care, discharge counseling, antimicrobial stewardship, and transitions of care. In addition, with increased enrollment and new accreditation standards, colleges and schools of pharmacy are faced with the need to have more quality experiential practice settings. With so many levels of students at different points in their experience, it becomes necessary to incorporate different teaching styles to maximize not only healthcare outcomes but student experiences, as well.

A LLM optimizes the use of student pharmacists and residents to provide patient care while improving the overall learning experience. The LLM consists of a team of pharmacists, pharmacy residents, and pharmacy students responsible for the patients' pharmaceutical care. This is similar to the traditional medical training model where the attending physician, residents, and students provide patient care. The attending pharmacist in the LLM is ultimately responsible for each patient while supervising other pharmacists, residents, and students.[10] The LLM allows for the pharmacists and residents to assume most of the responsibility for training the students, although models have been implemented that allow APPE students to provide pseudoprecepting for IPPE students, as well. For example, the PGY2 residents can oversee the learning of the PGY1 residents who then can oversee the learning of the APPE and IPPE students. This allows the attending pharmacist preceptor to focus on facilitating the overall responsibilities of the team. Examples of successful utilization of the LLM have been reported in the literature.[10-13] An example of a LLM for a transition of care program can be seen in Table 2-3.

Implementation of a LLM requires proper preplanning and buy-in from the entire pharmacy department. The department leaders should outline the goals and the anticipated patient-related outcomes for the program.

Suggested patient-related outcomes include:

- Identifying specific number of patient counseling encounters
- Identifying specific number of medication reconciliations completed
- Decrease in 30-day readmission rate
- Decrease in adverse drug reactions
- Decrease in cost of medications
- Improved use of medications
- Improvements in Hospital Consumer Assessment of Healthcare Providers and Systems scores

Planning should include identifying the practice areas targeted by the model and opportunities for future growth. The number of patients to be served, team make-up, role of team members, number of students, reporting lines, scheduling of activities, and measured outcomes should be determined with input from the staff and customized to your institution. The model should also be presented to colleges and schools of

Table 2-3. Layered Learning Model Example—Transition of Care	
Responsible Person	**Activity**
Pharmacy technician	Team informed of patient admission
IPPE student guided by APPE student	Obtain medication history from patient Patient discharge medications reviewed
APPE student guided by PGY1 resident	Any problems with medication orders resolved Medication problems resolved Any problems with discharge medications
PGY2 resident leads discussion	Medication regimen discussed by team
Preceptor	Assessment of learner skills
IPPE/APPE student guided by PGY1 resident	Discharge counseling provided
PGY1 resident guided by PGY2	Follow-up call to patient

pharmacy that would be sending students to the site. Ideally, the model will align with experiential program structure and student learning objectives (and avoid using students merely as cheap labor). Consideration for the type and number of learners a school can provide is crucial to the model's success. Health-system pharmacies may want to consider extending student placement opportunities to other schools outside the area if a single school cannot provide an adequate number of students for the program.

The increase in students assigned to the site may require a retooling of the first day's orientation program. You may consider creating a more structured orientation program to include site-specific onboarding and other important information or training to occur before starting the rotation. A designated point person or group of individuals should be directly responsible for orienting students. This helps to create an efficient and consistent process compared to requiring each preceptor to be responsible for his or her own orientation. The preceptors can then focus on providing the key information related to their practice and the specific rotation activities to assigned students.

LLM Challenges

Implementing a LLM will carry with it a number of key challenges such as the adequate coverage of the patient-care services when residents or students may not be present due to rotation schedules, holidays, weekends, and evenings. Consider alternative scheduling patterns with existing staff (such as paid pharmacy interns) and any available residents or students to help meet patient-care needs. The increase in students present on a service may also increase the number of individual assessments a preceptor may be responsible to complete. In these situations, the residents or other pharmacists on the team can be helpful in completing student evaluations, facilitating topic discussions, and assessing journal clubs or formal presentations. Because the preceptor is ultimately responsible for the team activities, you must balance the amount of oversight required for the team with providing one-on-one time with each student and resident.

One of the biggest challenges with the LLM is the potential to cause preceptor burnout. If you take on a significantly larger number of students than you can handle, the result will be unpleasant for both you and the students. To avoid burning out, you may want to consider enlisting residents, staff pharmacists, pharmacy technicians, and other supplemental preceptors to assist with the precepting. The school of pharmacy can help provide access to preceptor training for those staff who may be uncomfortable with the responsibility of precepting. By using others to help with precepting, you can gain free time to work on other responsibilities, develop colleagues' precepting skills, and ensure the students' positive learning experience. You may also want to take on a "divide and conquer" approach to multiple learners. Splitting the group across different parts of the institution will allow each trainee to maintain one-on-one time with you without creating a large, unwieldy entourage.

Though the LLM is an effective way to increase the impact of trainees on your practice site, there may be situations in which the LLM is not possible for the practice setting, such as an inadequate number of residents to make the model feasible to implement. Models for training students are not one-size-fits-all, and any model described in the literature will require significant customization to fit your practice.

Case Question

Starting in 3 months, SK will have responsibility for the following members of her team:

- *One full-time staff pharmacist responsible for medication distribution and limited clinical activities*
- *A PGY1 resident assigned three rotations for the year responsible for following all the patients on the service*
- *APPE students scheduled for 8-week acute care medicine blocks for 10 months of the year*
- *Two second-year pharmacy students assigned 2 days per week for 2-month blocks for their hospital IPPE*

How can SK best organize and manage a team of this size, maintain a transition of care program serving a floor of approximately 40 beds, and meet the residents' and pharmacy students' learning needs? What activities and responsibilities can she assign to each member of the team to maximize efficient use of the resources she has been provided?

> ## THE GIST

1. IPPEs provide pharmacy students the basic operational, professional, communication, and clinical skills in preparation for APPEs. The preceptor primarily provides the student direct instruction on essential skills needed for practice.
2. APPEs are intended to emphasize patient-centered care, medication therapy management, exposure to diverse patient populations, and delivery of care as part of an interprofessional team. The preceptor will spend less time on direct instruction and will, instead, provide more hands-on opportunities for the students to demonstrate their skills in performing these activities.
3. PGY1 pharmacy residencies provide the opportunity to further advance clinical practice skills, leadership, and project management skills. The preceptor's role is primarily to coach and facilitate as the residents learn how to take on the responsibilities of practicing pharmacists.
4. The PGY2 pharmacy residency largely focuses on a specific clinical pharmacy specialty practice. The residents should be afforded a high level of autonomy compared to a PGY1 resident or APPE student.
5. The LLM provides an opportunity for health systems to expand patient-care services while maintaining a beneficial experience for learners.

SUGGESTED READING

Cohen C, Dodd MA, Pandya DA et al. Fundamentals of experiential teaching. In Cuéllar LM, Ginsburg DB. *Preceptor's Handbook for Pharmacists*. 3rd ed. Bethesda, MD: ASHP; 2016.
 ◆ This chapter provides an overview of experiential programs in pharmacy schools. Examples of student activities for IPPEs and APPEs are provided.
Delgado O, Kernan WP, Knoer SJ. Advancing the pharmacy practice model in a community teaching hospital by expanding student rotations. *Am J Health-Syst Pharm*. 2014; 71:1871-76.
 ◆ This article describes the implementation and experience of a LLM community teaching model.

REFERENCES

1. Accreditation Council for Pharmacy Education. Accreditation standards and key elements for the professional program in pharmacy leading to the doctor of pharmacy degree. https://www.acpe-accredit.org/pdf/Standards2016FINAL.pdf. Accessed September 14, 2015.
2. Cuéllar LM, Ginsburg DB. *Preceptor's Handbook for Pharmacists*. 3rd ed. Bethesda MD: ASHP; 2016:85.

3. ASHP. ASHP accreditation standard for postgraduate year one (PGY1) pharmacy residency programs. http://www.ashp.org/DocLibrary/Accreditation/Newly-approved-PGY1-Standard-September-2014.pdf. Accessed September 14, 2015.
4. VARK: a guide to learning styles. 2014. www.vark-learn.com. Accessed February 28, 2016.
5. Kolb Learning Style Inventory (KLSI) 4.0. http://learningfromexperience.com/tools/kolb-learning-style-inventory-lsi/. Accessed February 28, 2016.
6. Lagasse C, Wilkinson S, Buck B et al. Integrating precepting into your daily practice. *Hosp Pharm.* 2013; 48:457-8.
7. ASHP. PGY2 outcomes, goals, and objectives. http://www.ashp.org/menu/Residency/Residency-Program-Directors/PGY2-Competency-Areas-Goals-and-Outcomes.aspx. Accessed February 28, 2016.
8. ASHP. ASHP accreditation standard for postgraduate year two (PGY2) pharmacy residency programs. http://www.ashp.org/DocLibrary/Accreditation/ASD-PGY2-Standard.aspx. Accessed September 14, 2015.
9. ASHP. Policies approved by the 2013 ASHP House of Delegates. http://www.ashp.org/DocLibrary/Policy/HOD/Officiallang2013Policies.aspx. Accessed September 14, 2015.
10. Delgado O, Kernan WP, Knoer SJ. Advancing the pharmacy practice model in a community teaching hospital by expanding student rotations. *Am J Health-Syst Pharm.* 2014; 71:1871-6.
11. Buie L. The layered learning practice model and the pharmacy practice model initiative. http://connect.ashp.org/browse/blogs/blogviewer?BlogKey=1ff0fea1-dd0b-46c3-81f6-b5c5ec1e0e95&ssopc=1&ct=584923c411a07b724316bb78f0eca4f6db cfac80aded2e578aabf5c90fd7807366eb6680d71d11d1e3ed5893f2718eeb66e6055 59e2328e49a794d0e45d11e13. Accessed September 14, 2015.
12. Chachine EB, El-Lababidi RM, Sourial M. Engaging pharmacy student, resident, and fellows in antimicrobial stewardship. *J Pharm Pract.* 2015; 28:585-91.
13. Soric MM, Glowczewski JE, Lerman RM. Implementing a layered learning model in a small community hospital: economic and patient satisfaction outcomes. *Am J Health-Syst Pharm.* 2016; 73:456-62.

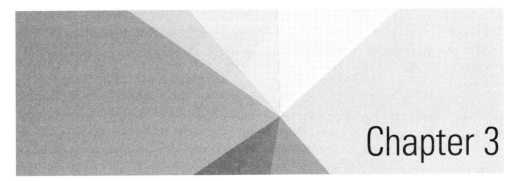

Chapter 3

Writing Your Syllabus or Learning Experience Description

Mate M. Soric

CASE STUDY

KS is a pharmacist in charge of running an internal medicine rotation for pharmacy residents. She has been running the rotation for a number of years and has received mixed reviews. Although some of her trainees love the experience and rave about the independence it offers, others complain about a lack of structure and being unfamiliar with the preceptor's expectations. Another year of rotations is about to begin, and KS is dreading the orientation session needed to get the next group of residents up to speed. She feels she regularly forgets some aspects of the orientation process and wishes it could be smoother this year.

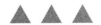

INTRODUCTION

Although it may not be a glamorous endeavor to put a syllabus together for a rotation, this document plays an incredibly important role in setting the stage for the learning experience, informing trainees of your expectations, and simplifying the orientation process. In addition to the obvious benefits to the learner, having a thorough syllabus offers significant benefits to the preceptor, as well. It can be used as a centralized location for commonly used instructions, limits repetitive explanations of assignments to learners, keeps orientation consistent, and serves as a repository for the rules and regulations that govern the entire experience.

THE PURPOSE OF A GOOD SYLLABUS OR LEARNING EXPERIENCE DESCRIPTION

Even though it may not always be readily apparent, learners truly appreciate a complete and organized syllabus.[1,2] Arriving on day one with clear expectations of the daily activities, the assessment plan, and what it takes to achieve a passing grade can go a long way to ease nerves. It is also a document that will serve as a reference throughout the experience, allowing learners to find answers when they encounter difficult situations or unclear expectations.

For the preceptor, a well-written syllabus can make your life a great deal easier. Referring your learners to the document can save you the time it would take to explain these activities time and time again. The syllabus also simplifies the orientation process by serving as a repository for the main points that should be reviewed with the trainees at the start of each rotation. By using the document as a guide, it means fewer facts and discussions will need to be memorized and recalled so you can focus your efforts elsewhere. Finally, by creating a one-stop shop for all of the rotation's rules and regulations, you limit the chance that an underperforming learner will plead ignorance when their grades are not as high as they would have liked.

Case Question

KS has identified an issue with residents consistently grasping her rotation's expectations. How could a written syllabus help standardize her rotation and orientation?

The terms *syllabus* and *learning experience description* throughout this chapter refer to a very similar document. A syllabus more often accompanies a student rotation and a learning experience description is the document that describes a resident's rotation. Because these documents often have significant overlap, we will use the term syllabus throughout the majority of the chapter. When describing sections that are specific to a residency learning experience description, that term will be used instead.

Quick Tip

Your syllabus is a dynamic document. After it is created, there is no reason that it cannot be changed or amended. As you encounter challenges, identify new learning opportunities, or see behaviors you would want to discourage, the syllabus should be updated, reworked, and amended to reflect the changing rotation it describes. Keeping the date of the last update in the footer of the document will help keep you up-to-date.

COMPONENTS OF THE SYLLABUS OR LEARNING EXPERIENCE DESCRIPTION

There are numerous organizational styles available for a rotation syllabus or a learning experience description. The precise format of your syllabus should be tailored to your rotation and precepting style. However, a sample syllabus is included in this text as a reference (see Appendix 3A).

Preceptor Contact

Taking a fairly prominent spot near the top of your syllabus, you should make it easy for your trainees to identify how to best contact you. The information you provide should identify the preferred method for communication in addition to some backup options. Typically, this includes email addresses, office phone, cellular phone, pager, and, sometimes, home phone numbers. If you are providing your personal contact information and you would like your residents and students to use them, make that clear in the document, as well. Most learners will hesitate to contact you on your home or personal cellular phone unless you have made it clear that you prefer that method. You may also consider including secondary preceptors or administrators that can be contacted in the event that you are unavailable. If you practice in an area susceptible to inclement weather, you may also want to establish a clear set of procedures for the trainee to communicate late arrivals or emergencies.

This section of the syllabus can also be used to describe the frequency, type, and extent of preceptor-learner interaction over the course of the rotation. This is a requirement for learning experience descriptions in residency programs and is greatly appreciated for student rotations, as well. Include the usual dates and times for scheduled rotation interactions, such as rounds, topic discussions or committee meetings, along with evaluations, presentations, and office hours.

General Description and Logistics

Although other sections included in this document will go into the rotation's details in greater degree, a brief introduction to the ins and outs of the experience should be placed near the top of the syllabus. It often opens with an overview of the kinds of experiences to which the learners will be exposed and highlights the general aspects of pharmacy practice that will be explored on the rotation. This section is also used to describe logistical concerns, such as parking, meeting location on the first day of the rotation, start and end times, lunch breaks, and navigation of the practice site. Many preceptors choose to include a map of the facility to help new learners get familiar with the lay of the land with clearly marked acceptable parking locations, meeting places, locations of restrooms, and food-friendly refrigerators and cafeterias.

You may also choose to include some tips to help incoming trainees prepare for the rotation so that they can hit the ground running and avoid remediation of important topics. For clinical rotations, you may consider including a list of disease states that the learners will routinely encounter. For other types of rotations, the list can include skills that the learner should review, such as spreadsheet software, pharmacy calculations, or a review of pharmacy laws that are pertinent to the practice site. If you have identified required readings that should be completed before the rotation begins, these should also be described here.

Quick Tip

If your rotation contains activities that occur during off-hours, make this expectation clear in the syllabus so that trainees are not caught off guard by these types of activities.

Attendance Policy

The syllabus is the ideal warehouse for the policies on learner attendance. If an emergency strikes, the trainees will already have access to this document and can refer to it to learn how to handle the situation appropriately. Ensure your attendance section discusses the difference between an excused and an unexcused absence. This will help limit inappropriate use of time off. A passage should also describe the procedures for notifying the preceptor or other stakeholders (such as the residency program director or the director of experiential education). To address instances where a learner will miss a significant amount of time, policies on family, sick, or professional leave should also be addressed, in addition to how supplemental assignments may be used to make up for lost time.

Quick Tip

You do not need to reinvent the wheel for each section of your syllabus. Chances are your residency program or the college or school of pharmacy sending you students has already created extensive policies and procedures on topics such as attendance and expectations. Feel free to use some of these existing statements as boilerplate language.

Goals, Objectives, and Activities

The goals, objectives, and activities that are expected to be evaluated during your rotation will most likely be handed down from the college or school of pharmacy sending you their students. For postgraduates, your residency program director will likely work with you to identify goals and objectives that should be assessed during your rotation. These learning objectives should also be clearly conveyed to the learners before they begin. As described in Chapter 1, a mapping activity should be completed to link the learning objectives to individual activities that the trainee will complete during the experience. A table such as the one provided in Chapter 1 (Table 1-2) is helpful to both the preceptor and the trainee. For the preceptor, completing the table will help identify the specific activities you will observe in order to assess each objective. For the learners, clear expectations of their day-to-day activities and how they relate to the final grade will help them prioritize their responsibilities and identify strengths and weaknesses effectively. Recall that it is particularly important to avoid using broad, general activities. Break up complex, multifaceted activities into smaller, bite-sized parts so that each component may be assessed. Instead of stating the learner will engage in "patient care," list activities such as collecting relevant patient data, identifying drug-related problems, creating a complete drug therapy plan, and implementing a monitoring plan.

Calendar

The portion of your syllabus that will be used most often will likely be the calendar. A detailed calendar that includes important deadlines, regularly scheduled activities, assessments, and preceptor availability is a great resource for your trainees and will be referenced throughout the experience. Although it may take a little extra work on your part as the preceptor, this document should be updated before each new rotation begins to allow for up-to-date information transmission to learners. For this reason, many preceptors are moving the calendar from paper to electronic formats. A single, unified online calendar allows all parties to edit and update the contents of the document so that everyone is seeing consistent information.

The Assessment Plan and Assignments

Your syllabus should contain a section that clearly describes to the learners how they will be evaluated and what acceptable performance looks like. It may be best to include a selection of common evaluation techniques that are used over the course of the rotation. If there are particular skills your rotation is best-suited to assess and improve, identify evaluations in these areas and when they are likely to be performed. Including actual copies of the rubrics used for these evaluations (such as presentation, journal club, or communication rubrics) will make expectations clear to the learners before they begin putting these projects together. You should also describe if and when a midpoint evaluation will be completed. If you use specific criteria to trigger a midpoint evaluation, those may also be described here.

When describing the final evaluation, a brief description of what it takes to earn each rating establishes expectations and minimizes confusion about grades. In particular, criteria should be laid out for what it takes to earn "honors," "A," or "achieved" marks. If there are certain behaviors or actions that would lead to an automatic failure of a rotation, the Assessment Plan section is the perfect place to communicate these consequences.

Even though you have described rotation activities earlier in the syllabus, you may also choose to include more detailed descriptions of projects and presentations in this section of the syllabus. For example, if you prefer that case presentations follow a certain format, including detailed instructions for that assignment in the syllabus is a significant benefit to your learners and to you. You can simply refer your students and residents to the syllabus for more detail and save yourself the time it takes to explain the assignment each month.

Expectations of Learner Progression

For resident learning experience descriptions, a section describing the expected progression over the course of the rotation is a requirement of the accreditation standard. A similar section could be useful for your students, although it is not a requirement for student rotations. It helps establish milestones for the trainees so that their self-evaluations can be based on your expectations and not on their own assumptions. Knowing your expectations will help struggling learners to seek out assistance before it is too late to correct the underlying issue. This section can be broken down into days or weeks and should specifically describe the types of activities and level of independence the learners should be achieving at various points in the experience. Ensure that the milestones are based on SMART (specific, measurable, attainable, realistic and timely) goals. If vague goals are used, the resident or student will not benefit from reading this section of your syllabus. For example, a clear expectation of learner progression could be written as "By the end of the first week of the rotation, students should be able to independently complete prescription transfers from outside pharmacies without direct preceptor involvement."

Case Question

KS's internal medicine rotation requires residents be independent in their patient work-up process by the end of the third week of the rotation. Write a SMART goal for inclusion in her learning experience description for this milestone.

DELIVERY OF THE SYLLABUS TO YOUR LEARNERS

It is best to plan to deliver your syllabus in advance of your learners' first day on your rotation. This advanced notice provides a chance for the learners to learn about the upcoming experience and begin working on any preparatory material before they arrive. Although it is in the learners' best interest to review the document before they arrive, this does not always occur. To increase the odds of getting your residents and students to read this important document, you can include your prerotation instructions in the syllabus and simply refer your incoming trainees to find their instructions within the syllabus rather than supplying them in the rotation's introductory email. This approach will decrease the time you spend providing instructions to incoming residents and students while having the added benefit of increasing the likelihood that the important details contained in the document reach their intended audience.

Case Question

KS has noticed that many of her residents are not actually reading the learning experience description she has prepared for them before they arrive for her rotation. Describe one strategy to increase the likelihood that they will do so.

▶ THE GIST

1. A syllabus is an important document for both learner and preceptor.
   a. It helps the learner be aware of the expectations of the experience.
   b. It helps minimize confusion and questions while promoting consistency.
2. A complete syllabus should contain contact information, the assessment plan, logistics, goals/objectives, a calendar, and the learners' expected progression.
3. To help ensure your learners read this important document, include all introductory information for your rotation in the syllabus and refer incoming learners to the document for instructions for day one.

SUGGESTED READING

Garavalia L, Hummel J, Wiley L, Huitt W. Constructing the course syllabus: faculty and student perceptions of important syllabus components. http://humphreys.edu/faculty/jdecosta/Jim/ED303/facultystudentperceptionssyllabus.pdf. Accessed 13 September 2016.

Gronlund NE. *How to Write and Use Instructional Objectives*. 7th ed. Upper Saddle River, NJ: Prentice Hall; 2004:3–29.

REFERENCES

1. O'Sullivan TA, Lau C, Patel M, Mac C et al. Student-valued measurable teaching behaviors of award-winning pharmacy preceptors. *Am J Pharm Educ*. 2015; 79:151.
2. Young S, Vos SS, Cantrell M, Shaw R. Factors associated with students' perception of preceptor excellence. *Am J Pharm Educ*. 2014; 78:53.

◆ APPENDIX 3A ◆

Sample Learning Experience Description

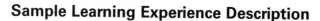

Advanced Internal Medicine I Rotation

Learning Experience Description

Preceptor Contact

Preceptor: John Smith, PharmD, BCPS

Office phone: 555-555-3037

Cell phone: 555-555-0398

Pager: 555-555-0900

Home phone: 555-555-8934

Email: john.smith@generalhospital.org

Preceptor Interaction

Daily:　8:00–8:30　　Pre rounds, Department of Pharmacy

　　　　8:30–11:30　Hospitalist team rounds (meet in ICU)

　　　　2:45–3:45　　Topic discussions

Tues:　1:30–2:30　　Office hours

Thurs:　9:45–11:45　Clinic

Preferred Communication

1. Daily scheduled meeting times
2. Email: Residents should check their email regularly (at least twice daily) as important communications may be sent via this route
3. Cell phone: Text message acceptable for non–patient care issues
4. Pager
5. Home phone: For emergencies only

General Description

Residents will round with the Hospitalist service, seeing approximately 15–30 patients per day, gaining skills in collecting and analyzing patient information, designing evidence-based drug regimens and monitoring plans, evaluating patient outcomes, and adjusting drug therapy in response to emerging data. In addition to the pharmacy resident, the Hospitalist team generally consists of an attending physician, a nurse practitioner, a clinical pharmacist, and pharmacy students on advanced pharmacy practice experience (APPE) rotations. Residents will also have the opportunity to provide education to patients, pharmacy students, nurses, and physicians. Emphasis will be placed

Source: Adapted from ASHP's Residency Program Design and Conduct (RPDC) Workshops. Used with permission ©ASHP, Bethesda, MD. http://www.ashp.org/DocLibrary/Accreditation/ Learning-Experience-Description-Example-New-2014-PGY1-Standard.pdf

on evaluation of medical literature, communication skills, and the development of a commitment to lifelong learning. In addition to the requirements outlined above, the Advanced Internal Medicine I rotation will allow the resident to serve as a preceptor for an APPE pharmacy student. Additional responsibilities may include syllabus creation, formative evaluations, summative evaluation, and project assignment/assessment of an APPE student.

Location, Lunch, and Parking

General Hospital is located at 1234 Main Street, Cleveland, OH 44102. With 430 beds, it is the largest community hospital in the health system. A cafeteria is available onsite; however, a refrigerator is available if a student prefers to pack a lunch. Parking is free for residents in Lot B.

Disease States

It may be worthwhile to review some of the common disease states seen on the Internal Medicine rotation before your rotation begins, such as:

Cardiology

- Acute coronary syndromes
- Congestive heart failure
- Hypertension
- Hyperlipidemia
- Atrial fibrillation
- Stroke

Endocrine

- Diabetes mellitus
- Hyper/hypothyroidism

Gastroenterology

- Gastroesophageal reflux disease
- Peptic ulcer disease
- Pancreatitis
- Hepatitis

Infectious Disease

- Pneumonia
- Urinary tract infections
- Skin and soft tissue infections
- Infective endocarditis
- Sepsis

Nephrology

- Acute and chronic renal failure
- Drug-induced renal failure

Neurology/Psychiatry

- Pain management
- Depression

- Dementia
- Drug and alcohol withdrawal

Pulmonology

- Chronic obstructive pulmonary disease
- Asthma

Throughout the course of the rotation, the resident will be expected to gain proficiency for common disease states through direct patient care and educational offerings for students and other healthcare professionals.

Topic Discussions

Topic discussions are designed to:

- provide a review of selected disease states or conditions.
- practice small-group presentation skills.

Topic discussions are assigned weekly (one per learner) and typically delivered at the end of the day.

Assignment

1. Choose a topic that fits with the week's theme and submit it to Dr. Smith for approval.
2. Review your class notes, guidelines, and pertinent primary literature to design a 30–45 min presentation on the assigned topic.
   a. Focus on the areas of pathophysiology, clinical presentation, treatment, and monitoring.
   b. Other components may be included as you see fit.
   c. Do not overlook recent developments (i.e., what has changed since you had your lecture in pharmacy school).
3. Create a complete, yet succinct, handout for your audience.
4. Deliver your presentation using your best presentation skills.
   a. Please do not read your handout to the audience! Deliver your presentation in the style that you would like to see a presentation given.
   b. Stick to the time limits.
   c. Practice ahead of time, if necessary.

Journal Club

Journal club assignments are designed to:

- evaluate the learner's evidence-based medicine skills.
- identify emerging evidence that might be of use to practicing pharmacists.
- examine studies closely for strengths and weakness to determine the clinical applicability of the data published.

Assignment

1. Choose a recent journal article of interest to you.
   a. It may be from any area of interest.
   b. It should be recent (from the last 2 yr or so).
   c. Most likely it will be a randomized control trial, although others may be accepted after review.

2. Email the article to Dr. Smith for approval.
3. Once approved, you may begin the preparation of a journal club handout.
   a. Typically, a Power Point presentation is not necessary, although it may be done if you prefer this delivery method.
   b. If needed, Dr. Smith has a number of sample handouts for you to review.
4. Email an electronic copy of the journal article to all likely attendees of the journal club.
   a. This includes pharmacists, residents, and other students.
   b. All attendees are expected to come prepared to participate in the journal club.
5. On the day of the presentation, arrive prepared with handouts for all likely attendees.

General Handout Structure

Background: Current gold standard of practice for the disease state, condition, or medication described in the article. Brief description of any other relevant trials

Methods: The plan for the design and implementation of the study. Includes study design, inclusion/exclusion criteria, primary and secondary endpoints, study protocol, statistical analysis, and funding (including the role of the sponsor).

Results: Baseline population characteristics, primary endpoints and those secondary endpoints that raise important clinical questions that should be answered by a study of their own. Should include both measures of statistical significance and, when possible, clinical significance.

Author's Conclusion: Paraphrased from the article.

Critique: Strengths and weaknesses of the trial.

Your Conclusions: Rewritten conclusion statement that accurately reflects what a practicing pharmacist can take from the trial.

Unanswered Questions: What questions were left unanswered by the trial (or were raised by) the trial.

References: Written in proper format.

Goals and Objectives to Be Taught and Formally Evaluated

During the learning experience the resident will focus on the goals and objectives outlined below by performing the activities that are associated with each objective. The resident will gradually assume responsibility for all of the patients within the assigned unit. The postgraduate year 1 resident must devise efficient strategies for accomplishing the required activities in a limited time frame. Achievement of the goals of the residency is determined through assessment of ability to perform the associated objectives. The table below demonstrates the relationship between the activities and the goals/objectives assigned to the learning experience.

Competency Area R1: Patient Care		
Goal R1.1: In collaboration with the healthcare team, provide safe and effective patient care to a diverse range of patients, including those with multiple comorbidities, high-risk medication regimens, and multiple medications following a consistent patient care process.		
R1.1.1	(Applying) Interact effectively with healthcare teams to manage patients' medication therapy.	Actively participate in daily hospitalist team rounds. ♦ Establish a strong rapport with the other members of the hospitalist team ♦ Communicate recommendations effectively to the team Provide drug information for patients, caregivers, and/or healthcare providers
R1.1.2	(Analyzing) Collect information on which to base safe and effective medication therapy.	Accurately and efficiently gather patient information from the electronic medical record and analyze it to: ♦ Prioritize the patient's medical problems ♦ Identify all drug-related problems
R1.1.3	(Creating) Design or redesign safe and effective patient-centered therapeutic regimens and monitoring plans (care plans).	Design a complete patient care plan that is customized to each patient's unique situation, including: ♦ Therapeutic goals ♦ Complete therapeutic recommendations that include drug, dose, route, frequency and duration ♦ Monitoring parameters for both efficacy and safety ♦ Important patient education topics Complete formal consults for the pharmacy consult service, including pain management, polypharmacy, discharge education, anticoagulation and renal dosing.

(continued)

R1.1.4	(Applying) Ensure implementation of therapeutic regimens and monitoring plans (care plans) by taking appropriate follow-up actions.	Complete formal consults for the pharmacy consult service, including pain management, polypharmacy, discharge education, anticoagulation and renal dosing. Follow up on previous recommendations to ensure continued appropriateness
R1.1.5	(Applying) Document direct patient care activities appropriately in the medical record or where appropriate.	Document all patient care and medication education-related activities in subjective, objective, assessment, and plan (SOAP) note format in the patient's medical record.
R1.1.6	(Applying) Demonstrate responsibility to patients.	Prioritize responsibilities to allow for completion of patient care activities.

Competency Area R2: Teaching, Education, and Dissemination of Knowledge

Goal R2.1: Provide effective medication and practice-related education to patients, caregivers, healthcare professionals, students, and the public (individuals and groups).

R2.1.1	(Applying) Design effective educational activities.	Participate in (and often lead) daily topic discussions with APPE students, including the preparation and evaluation of handouts, journal clubs, and continuing pharmacy education presentations. Use case-based teaching to convey important therapeutics topics to pharmacy students.
R2.1.2	(Applying) Use effective presentation and teaching skills to deliver education.	Serve as the primary preceptor for at least one pharmacy student, creating a syllabus, organizing learning experiences and evaluating the student appropriately.
R2.1.3	(Applying) Appropriately assess effectiveness of education.	Serve as the primary preceptor for at least one pharmacy student, creating a syllabus, organizing learning experiences, and evaluating the student appropriately.

(continued)

Goal R2.2: Effectively employ appropriate preceptors' roles when engaged in teaching (e.g., students, pharmacy technicians, or other healthcare professionals).		
R2.2.1	(Analyzing) When engaged in teaching, select a preceptors' role that meets learners' educational needs.	Serve as the primary preceptor for at least one pharmacy student, creating a syllabus, organizing learning experiences and evaluating the student appropriately. Choose the appropriate preceptor role based on student experience, comfort, knowledge base and other factors.
R2.2.2	(Applying) Effectively employ preceptor roles, as appropriate.	Serve as the primary preceptor for at least one pharmacy student, creating a syllabus, organizing learning experiences and evaluating the student appropriately. Depending on the situation, employ the four preceptor roles to effectively provide experiential education to pharmacy students.

Expected Progression of Resident Responsibilities

The length of time specified below represents a general estimation and will be customized based on the resident's abilities and timing of the learning experience during the year.

Day 1: Orientation to the learning experience, expectation discussions and goal-setting.

Week 1: The resident will continue to improve their patient evaluation and problem identification skills along with the added responsibility of precepting an APPE student. An initial rapport will be established with the pharmacy student during the first week.

Weeks 2–3: Additional focus will be placed on the design and communication of the therapeutic regimen. The preceptor will begin to shift toward a facilitator's role as the resident demonstrates an ability to make sound recommendations with all relevant evidence to increase the likelihood of acceptance by the team. He will attend rounds on an occasional basis. The resident's interaction with the students will be assessed, including any formative evaluations, topic discussion sessions, and other assigned student work.

Week 4: A summative evaluation will take place that encompasses the clinical aspects of the rotation (focusing on problem identification, plan design, and plan communication) along with the resident's ability to incorporate a student pharmacist into his or her practice.

Evaluation Strategy

Throughout the rotation, the preceptor will provide an opportunity for the resident to practice and document formative self-assessment in addition to the preceptor's ongoing formative assessments. At the end of the rotation, the preceptor will complete a summative assessment of the pharmacy resident. The pharmacy resident, preceptor, and residency program director will review and make comment on this evaluation. The pharmacy resident will complete a self-evaluation and an evaluation of each learning experience and each rotation preceptor. Resident evaluation meetings may be scheduled more frequently if the resident or faculty identifies areas of concern. Academic or professional performance requiring corrective action will be handled using the policies and procedures set forth in General Hospitals' Policies and Procedures and the Residency Handbook.

What	Snapshot	Who	When
Formative	Developing a therapeutic plan	Preceptor	End of Week 2
Formative self-evaluation	Developing a therapeutic plan	Resident	End of Week 2
Formative	Grading a Student	Preceptor	End of Week 4
Formative self-evaluation	Grading a Student	Resident	End of Week 4
Summative (optional)		Preceptor	Midpoint
Summative self-evaluation (optional)		Resident	Midpoint
Summative		Preceptor	End of each learning experience
Summative self-evaluation		Resident	End of each learning experience
Preceptor evaluation		Resident	End of each learning experience
Learning experience evaluation		Resident	End of each learning experience

Calendar of Events

Sun	Mon	Tue	Wed	Thu	Fri	Sat
3	4 **Rotation Begins** 8:00 - Orientation 9:00 - Rounds 10:00 - Warfarin Education 2:45 - Topic Discussion	5 8:00 - Rounds 2:45 - Topic Discussion	6 8:00 - Rounds 2:45 - Topic Discussion	7 8:00 - Rounds 10:00 - Clinic 2:45 - Topic Discussion	8 8:00 - Rounds 2:45 - Topic Discussion	9
10	11 8:00 - Rounds 10:00 - Warfarin Education 3:00 - Topic Discussion	12 8:00 - Rounds 3:00 - Topic Discussion	13 8:00 - Rounds 10:00 - Feedback Session 3:00 - Topic Discussion	14 8:00 - Rounds 10:00 - Clinic 3:00 - Topic Discussion	15 8:00 - Rounds 3:00 - Topic Discussion	16
17	18 **Dr. S. Offsite** MLK Day 8:00 - Rounds 10:00 - Warfarin Education 3:00 - Topic Discussion	19 8:00 - Rounds 1:00 - Journal Club 3:00 - Topic Discussion	20 8:00 - Rounds 3:00 - Topic Discussion	21 8:00 - Rounds 10:00 - Clinic 3:00 - Topic Discussion	22 8:00 - Rounds 10:00 - Feedback Session 3:00 - Topic Discussion	23
24	25 8:00 - Rounds 10:00 - Warfarin Education 3:00 - Topic Discussion	26 8:00 - Rounds 3:00 - Topic Discussion	27 8:00 - Rounds 3:00 - Topic Discussion	28 8:00 - Rounds 10:00 - Clinic 1:00 - Feedback Session 3:00 - Topic Discussion	29 8:00 - Rounds 2:00 - Final Evaluation	30

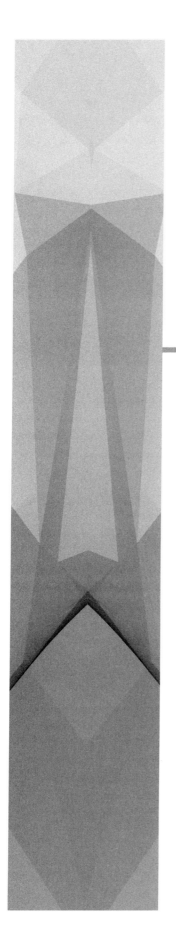

Part II

Conducting the
Experience

4. Orientation 47
    Mate M. Soric

5. The Art of Teaching 55
    Stacey R. Schneider

6. Assessing Learner Performance 69
    S. Scott Wisneski

7. Dealing with Difficult Situations 87
    Stacey R. Schneider

8. Wrapping Up the Rotation 105
    S. Scott Wisneski

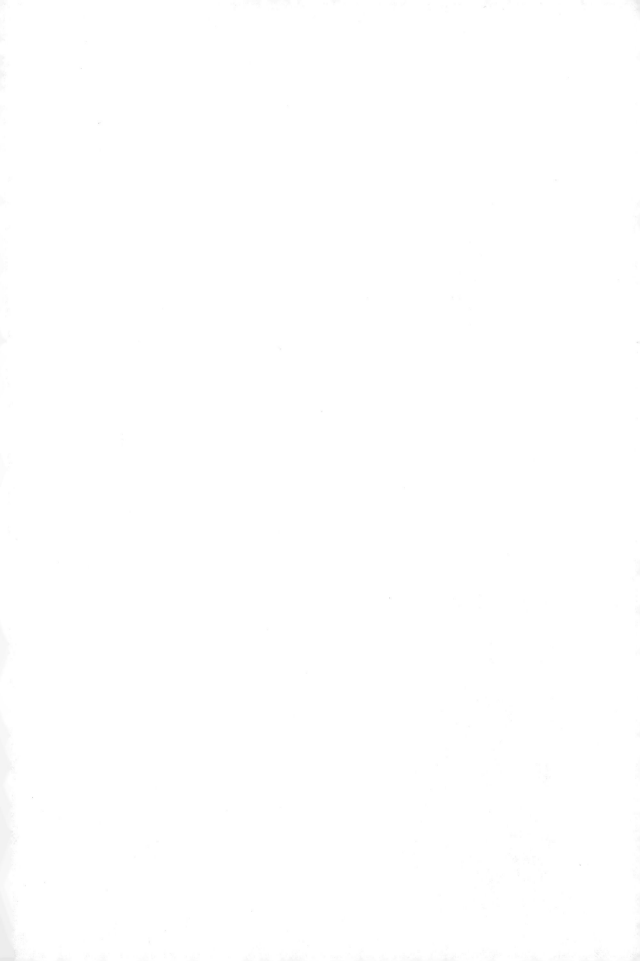

Chapter 4

Orientation

Mate M. Soric

CASE STUDY

RC is a new preceptor for a cardiology rotation at a large academic medical center. He has taken his colleague's advice and has developed a syllabus for his rotation that has been sent along to his first group of students before their arrival. The first day of the rotation begins in just a few hours, but RC has not considered what it takes to move from the planning stages of the rotation to actually getting the students up and running on the first day.

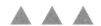

SYLLABUS REVIEW AND EXPECTATION DISCUSSIONS

As discussed in Chapter 3, a great deal of planning and time should be invested in a rotation syllabus. The document should stand alone as a clear set of expectations and responsibilities for the rotation and is, ideally, sent out to the learners before their first day of rotation. On day one of the experience, however, it may be wise to avoid assuming its target audience has studied the document in great detail. For this reason, the orientation period for your learning experience should include a syllabus review and a discussion of the learner's expectations. Reviewing this information face-to-face with your trainees can help clear up misunderstandings for those who have read the document and provide the first glimpse of the ins and outs of the rotation for those who have not yet had a chance to dive into the syllabus.

Typically, the orientation discussions can open with a review of the day-to-day activities the learner will be required to complete. Take time to highlight the order of events for a normal day and any exceptions to this established schedule. If you will be assigning longitudinal projects, let the trainees know at the beginning of the experience so that they can manage their time more effectively. As you are reviewing the day-to-day activities, a discussion of the assessment criteria will likely follow. Much in the same way you matched activities to learning objectives (as described in Chapter 1), it helps to describe these linkages to the students or residents. In this way, they will know exactly how they will be evaluated for each activity in the rotation. If there are certain performance indicators that you use to assign an "A" or "honors" grade, share these with the trainees upfront.

You may have a sense of how a "star" student would perform on your rotation, including their:

♦ Interactions with patients, caregivers, and providers
♦ Drug and disease state knowledge
♦ Application of knowledge base to patient care or other scenarios

You should share these expectations with your learners during orientation so you don't leave them in the dark about how to achieve success. Similarly, if there are behaviors that would act as a barrier to high-quality student or resident performance, be forthcoming about those, as well.

Behaviors that would result in an automatic dismissal should be included in this list, such as:

♦ Professionalism issues (including dress, behavior, use of technology, etc.)
♦ Disclosing protected health information
♦ Causing patient harm

Case Question

RC has put a great deal of work into his syllabus and provided it to his incoming students before they arrive onsite. Why is it beneficial to schedule additional rotation time to review the document face-to-face with learners?

TRAINING AND LOGISTICS

The early portions of a rotation are bound to be filled with various bits of paperwork, meet and greets, and new employee training. Although there is little academic value in most of these activities, there is no better time to get these requirements out of the way than in the orientation period. To help your trainees get acclimated to the practice site, a tour of the facility should be completed that includes all of the areas in which the students or residents will be expected to work. Be sure to identify restrooms, workspaces, and the appropriate locations to store and eat meals. As you usher the learners around the facility, introduce them to your colleagues, especially those they will be encountering on a daily basis. If the human resources department at your practice site has onboarding requirements, set aside time to complete any mandatory training, obtain name badges, or gain computer access.

The importance of pharmacy information systems (such as electronic medical records or dispensing software) has never been greater. In nearly every practice environment, trainees will rely on these systems to gather pertinent information and provide patient care. For this reason, ensure that you are earmarking a significant amount of time to orient learners to these systems. Consider including a modeling session with your learners in which you talk through your thought process as you complete the kinds of activities that the students or residents will also be asked to complete. For example, in a clinical setting, working up a patient as a group can help shed light on common shortcuts and efficiencies that may be second nature for you but would not be intuitive for someone unfamiliar with the system. If an inadequate amount of time is spent on this vital part of the orientation process, you risk negatively affecting all other aspects of the rotation that rely on the proper use of the pharmacy information system.

Case Question

RC's first students are onsite and struggling to work up the amount of patients that he had expected. Although the students tend to catch most of the important information, it is taking them significantly longer than RC expected to navigate the electronic medical record. How could RC allow for a smoother transition to a new system for his trainees?

GETTING TO KNOW THE LEARNER

Thus far, the majority of the discussion has come from the preceptor communicating the expectations of the rotation to the learners. These discussions are important for establishing a good student-preceptor relationship, but you want to exercise care to avoid commandeering the entire orientation. In the end, more time should be spent listening to the learners than is spent lecturing to them. After all, the orientation is just as much a chance to learn about the learners' needs, experiences, and capabilities as it is a chance to expound on the contents of your syllabus. You have a number of tools at your disposal to collect information on your trainees to help you shape their learning experience.

Portfolio or Curriculum Vitae Review

Before learners arrive for your rotation, you may have access to a portfolio or curriculum vitae. The data contained in these documents are a good starting point as you get a feel for the trainees' previous experiences and how they may affect your rotation. Even though this information is readily available, be careful to avoid relying solely on these documents. They are a general description of the types of experiences the trainees have had thus far, but they do not speak to the quality of the experiences. Ideally, these documents will serve as a first step toward understanding your learners' needs.

Discussions with the Learner

The most readily available source of information will likely be the trainees, themselves. Simply asking them about their career aspirations, what they hope to gain by completing your rotation, their biggest strengths and weaknesses, and other rotations they have completed or plan to complete can help you understand the adjustments that might be necessary for each learner. This information may not always be complete or unbiased, but it certainly provides an excellent starting point.

Previous Evaluations

Unless you are the first rotation scheduled for a given trainee, a wealth of information on past performance can be uncovered by reading previous evaluations. However, due to student privacy laws, you may not have access to all of the students' previous evaluations. Some colleges and schools of pharmacy withhold all of this information, whereas others may provide a snapshot of the students' previous rotations. For residents, previous resident performance is often a topic of discussion at residency advisory committee meetings. The residency program director can choose to share summative evaluations with other preceptors in an effort to coordinate educational opportunities and correct deficiencies. If you have this information available to you, use it to appropriately shape your learning experience to better fit the learners who will be completing it. For example, if previous preceptors have consistently identified an area of weakness, consider customizing your rotation to emphasize that practice area. Alternatively, if a number of preceptors have identified an objective as achieved, you can move some of your attention away from that objective in favor of others not yet achieved. One important caveat to the use of previous evaluations: avoid becoming biased toward a learner based on the contents of previous evaluations. Always complete your own objective assessment of your learners and supplement the information found in past evaluations with information gathered during your rotation.

Quick Tip

If the college or school of pharmacy in your area does not offer information from past rotations, you can still try to tap into this valuable knowledge by asking the students directly. Their assessment of their own progress may not be as objective as those from other preceptors, but it can still be a good starting point for future customization of the rotation.

Baseline Testing

One way to gather an objective measurement of the learners' knowledge base is to create a standard baseline examination of topics that are commonly encountered on your rotation. A number of resources can be used to help you create the test, such as board preparation texts, top 200 drug lists, or exams created by other pharmacists for similar rotations. If you are unfamiliar with the tenets of test writing, it may be best to use an established exam to avoid some of the pitfalls of writing poor exam items.[1] Regardless of the source of the examination, ensure it contains a mix of entry-level and advanced topics from different aspects of your practice so that the depth as well as breadth of trainee knowledge is assessed. A short amount of time can be set aside during the orientation to allow the learners to complete the examinations and allow for the preceptor to grade them. The examinations can be low stakes (meaning the score has no impact on final grade) and still be used to collect valuable information on the types of knowledge gaps. If it is coupled with a final examination at the end of the learning experience, the grades on the two examinations can be used as an objective measurement of learners' progression over the course of the rotation.

Quick Tip

You should discuss the findings of the examination with the learners so that a mutually agreed-upon plan can be put in place to correct knowledge gaps. To avoid the students sharing the contents with others, you should keep the hard copy of the examination.

Direct Observation

Some skills may be difficult to evaluate in previous evaluations or paper tests, especially tasks that may be unique to your practice site or based on soft skills. If learners are expected to perform high-level duties independently on your rotation, you may also want more concrete evidence that the learners are up to the task. In these cases, it may be best to include an opportunity for the learners to observe the proper execution of the task and then perform the task under the direct supervision of the preceptor. By directly supervising the learners during the orientation period, the preceptor can provide a sign-off before the trainees are allowed to perform independently. The data gathered during these direct observations are real time, not subject to differing expectations among preceptors, and can evaluate application of knowledge in addition to the recall of facts. To make these observation sessions even more useful (to you and your students or residents), consider creating a rubric for the activities that will be observed. This helps standardize your assessments and provides a clear set of expectations to your trainees before the observation period begins.

Case Question

RC asks his students to counsel patients at discharge on the indication and side effects of their new medications. He has had issues with students scaring patients with long lists of side effects, leading to nonadherence to the new medications. How could RC ensure that all his students are providing this counseling in a manner that is consistent with his expectations?

Quick Tip

You may find it helpful to create a file for each trainee on rotation. Use the file to keep track of student expectations, examinations, rubrics, and any other data you collect over the course of the rotation (especially if you are juggling multiple learners at the same time). Hard copies of rubrics are much more useful at final evaluation time than fading memories of trainee performance.

Customizing the Rotation

The purpose of all this data collection is to identify the unique needs of each of your learners, but it does not mean that you need to reinvent your entire learning experience each time a new batch of learners arrives. Using the process identified earlier (see Chapter 1), it is beneficial to establish a core set of rotation activities, assessments, and learning opportunities that remain fairly consistent from rotation to rotation. To set your learning experience in stone, however, would also be a mistake, because each learner has a different set of needs. The ideal rotation will contain customizable aspects to help ensure the learners obtain the kinds of experiences that will help them reach their career goals and improve on their personal weaknesses. It is beneficial to identify a number of easily customizable activities and experiences that can be tweaked for each new round of trainees that are on-site.

Some examples of easily customizable aspects of the experience include:

♦ Type of formative assessments completed for each learner
♦ Presence or absence of a midpoint summative evaluation
♦ Use of elective learning objectives
♦ Use of supplemental preceptors
♦ Longitudinal projects

The orientation itself is an important customizable aspect of the rotation. For instance, you may uncover that you have a student on rotation with a long history of working in your practice setting. In these cases, the orientation may be shortened or focused on higher-level skills that the student still needs to learn. On the other hand, you may also identify a student that has never set foot in your practice setting and may require additional orientation that might not be standard for your typical student population.

> ## *Case Question*
>
> *RC has a student onsite this month who has spent a number of years completing medication reconciliation in an emergency department setting. The student has not, however, spent any time providing patient counseling on cardiac medications. How might this previous experience impact the rotation orientation, which typically includes a full day shadowing technicians completing medication reconciliation on the cardiology unit and a day with a resident completing counseling activities?*

You may also consider customizing the delivery of your learning material based on the learning style of the students that you precept. In general, learning styles remain a controversial area of educational theory. There are a number of different instruments and surveys that can be utilized to help with the identification of preferences, but many are not validated, and no established list of education styles exists.[2] Some feel that always aligning your teaching style with that of your learners deprives them of the chance to learn to adapt to various teaching styles. Therefore, it may be beneficial to consider learning styles when you are attempting to deliver educational material, but are failing to connect with your audience. Consider varying the way you deliver this material over the course of the rotation with a mixture of lectures, application activities, diagrams or drawings, and other methods.

You may also encounter generational differences in expectations and attitudes that lead to misunderstandings or other miscues between you and your learners. These kinds of issues highlight the importance of clear expectations and a solid orientation for all learners. If you encounter recurring problems, you may want to update the syllabus and orientation discussions to cover these topics. If the problems stem from communication issues, you can survey students or residents who have completed the rotation to identify exactly where the disconnect occurred and remedy the problem for future rotations.

EASING THE BURDEN OF ORIENTATION

Considering all of the aspects of an effective orientation described in this chapter, it becomes clear that proper orientation is a time-consuming endeavor. Because the typical preceptor has multiple responsibilities that need to be completed in addition to their precepting duties, it is fairly easy to see how orientation is often sacrificed when competing requirements conflict. If you see a quality orientation as an investment into a smooth, problem-free rotation, you will conclude that it is time well spent. There are a number of ways to maintain the quality of the orientation and still save considerable amounts of time.

A number of lecture capture products are available (PowerPoint, Camtasia, Jing, etc.) that can be used to record the standard contents of an orientation session. The syllabus review, daily activities, grading discussion, and attendance policies are not likely to change significantly from rotation to rotation and can be covered in such a video. Preceptors can assign video viewing to occur before trainees officially begin their rotation to streamline the on-boarding process and increase the time available for other activities. This approach to simplifying orientation will not completely replace the traditional orientation experience, but it does allow the focus to turn to the learners and away from the preceptor. If aspects of the rotation do change over time, be sure you update your orientation videos accordingly or the information you are sharing may do more harm than good.

If you are taking multiple learners over the course of the year, you can attempt to stagger start times (especially for 6- to 8-week rotations) to allow established learners to take part in the orientation of incoming learners. Instead of the preceptor providing modeling, the seasoned learners can step in and demonstrate the proper way to complete rotation activities or use the pharmacy information systems. If your rotations do not allow for this type of staggering (for those with set start and end dates or shorter rotations), consider utilizing residents that are available at your institution as preceptor extenders. Conducting an effective orientation process is a valuable learning experience for the residents that will one day be taking students of their own, and, at the same time, it frees up the preceptor to attend to other duties.

▶ THE GIST

1. Orientation is a critical part of a good rotation.
2. The length and depth of orientation can be customized to the learner.
3. It helps to review key components of the syllabus with students to ensure understanding.
4. A significant portion of the orientation period should allow the preceptor to get to know the learners so that the rotation can be shaped to meet their needs.
5. Orientation can be time-consuming, therefore, it may be beneficial to enlist the help of other learners to complete some of the components described in this chapter.

SUGGESTED READING

Sheaffer SL, DeRemer CE, Yam NT. Precepting fundamentals. In: Cuéllar LM, Ginsburg DB, eds. *Preceptor's Handbook for Pharmacists*. 3rd ed. Bethesda, MD: ASHP; 2016:1-20.

REFERENCES

1. Kelley KA. What Matters in Assessment? In: Sylvia LM, Barr JT, eds. *Pharmacy Education: What Matters in Teaching and Learning*. Sudbury, MD: Jones and Bartlett; 2011:85-101.
2. Cassidy S. Learning styles: an overview of theories, models, and measures. *Educ Psychol*. 2004; 24:419-44.

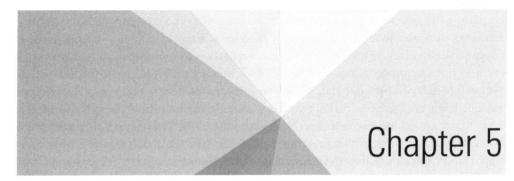

The Art of Teaching

Stacey R. Schneider

CASE STUDY

JK is a new preceptor at a clinical ambulatory care site and has been asked by her supervisor to create a teaching philosophy. She has been assigned one advanced pharmacy practice experience (APPE) student and one resident to precept for 2 months. Her supervisor has encouraged her to use this time to reflect on her teaching style and requests the document at the end of the 2-month timeframe. She has never prepared a document like this before and has no idea how to begin.

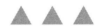

INTRODUCTION

So many of us begin teaching careers with little training and continue with intermittent moments of professional development to enhance our teaching skills. The method you choose to deliver information to your learners reflects your own experiences in the teaching and learning process. You will be faced with many different types of learners, and you will need to adjust your style to deliver information effectively. You will encounter various levels of desire for learning, and it is a challenge to nurture an environment that fosters excitement for learning. Teaching is an interaction between an instructor and a student, thus the impact of this relationship rather than the activity itself is of primary importance. Continual improvement in teaching requires ongoing reflection on your own along with the assessment of student learning.

WRITING A TEACHING PHILOSOPHY

Every teacher has a philosophy of teaching whether he or she realizes it or not. Defined simply, a *philosophy of teaching* is the conceptualization of your teaching and learning process. Consider your thoughts and beliefs about how learning occurs and how your teaching style will facilitate future learning. Determine how those beliefs will translate into action in your practice environment. Consider your students' needs and how you will address those needs. Allowing your learners to understand your perspective on your role as a teacher will help them understand your expectations. A teaching philosophy is a kind of personal mission statement for those who are committed to teaching. It helps to communicate your goals to the learner and demonstrates that you are thoughtful and reflective in your teaching approach.

There is no set format for writing a teaching philosophy. It is generally one to two pages in length and written in the first-person and present tense. Your philosophy should set you apart from others. It should create a vivid impression of a teacher who demonstrates a unique approach and commitment to the art of teaching. Include specific examples of teaching strategies so the reader will be able to visualize the learning environment you wish to create. You may start by determining exactly what you expect students to master by the end of the rotation. Imagine how to facilitate student learning so that every student has the opportunity to reach this level. This perspective implies that you can articulate specific learning goals, develop assessments that measure these goals, and have a support structure to allow all students to master this level of learning.

Quick Tip

Think about teachers who have influenced you (both negatively and positively) with their teaching styles as you begin to put your own teaching philosophy on paper.

The key elements to a teaching philosophy usually include your learning goals for your students, teaching methods, assessment of student learning, and assessment of your teaching abilities.

The following are a few questions that may help you to explore your teaching style and crystallize your thoughts into a formal philosophy:

♦   What do you hope students will appreciate about your practice environment?
♦   How do you view the relationship between the teacher and the learner?
♦   What assessment tools do you use (e.g., tests, reflections, active learning strategies)?
♦   What are your strengths as a teacher?

A 2011 *Advances in Physiology Education* article by Kearns and Sullivan[1] provides more information and suggestions.

A teaching philosophy is a living document that will evolve over time. Active reflection on your philosophy is required for continued renewal of your goals and teaching methods. Consider this document as you would your curriculum vitae, reflecting your growth as both a teacher and a healthcare professional. It will provide you with a road map to document your strengths and identify areas for further improvement. The teaching philosophy can provide an opportunity for you to formulate your personal and professional career objectives and guide your future plans. See Box 5-1 for a sample teaching philosophy.

Case Question

After hosting her first rotation and reflecting on her own experiences as a learner, JK has formulated the teaching philosophy in Box 5-1. How has JK addressed the learning goals for her students, teaching methods, assessment of student learning, and assessment of her own teaching abilities in the teaching philosophy?

PRECEPTOR ROLES

Preceptors will encounter many different kinds of students with diverse learning needs in the clinical environment. For this reason, preceptors are required to be skilled in multiple roles to best serve the individual learner's needs. ASHP has advocated ongoing efforts to develop the skills of clinicians serving as preceptors to residents and students. This model of teaching clinical problem solving is meant to foster cognitive learning.

The process of cognitive learning has been divided into six levels:

1.   Obtaining knowledge
2.   Comprehending the knowledge
3.   Applying the knowledge
4.   Analyzing the clinical problem
5.   Synthesizing an answer to the clinical problem
6.   Evaluating the end result

A learner may present at any of these stages. There are four different roles a preceptor can assume depending on the individual student's needs: direct instruction, modeling, coaching, and facilitating.[2]

Direct instruction occurs when the preceptor conveys knowledge directly to the learner using lectures, discussions, or assigned readings. This type of instruction is

BOX 5-1. SAMPLE TEACHING PHILOSOPHY

I am a novice as a teacher in a professional environment new to me. My goal is to participate in preparing students to practice as a generalist within the healthcare system. To be a successful practitioner, one must possess the values of honesty, integrity, and professionalism at all times. The primary responsibility of a pharmacist is to ensure optimal delivery of safe and effective medications and be an integral part of the healthcare team. The knowledge and skills gained at this site will help the student to display excellent communication skills with both patients and colleagues and prepare them for practice with an interprofessional team.

It is my responsibility to create a student-centered learning environment that fosters the development of critical thinking and lifelong learning. My primary goal at every interaction is to ensure the atmosphere is comfortable and the material presented is engaging. I believe that a teacher must have passion for the material to ignite in the student an enthusiasm to learn. I believe students will come and participate if I can develop a session in which they are excited about learning and feel comfortable no matter what stage of learning is taking place. Sessions that involve active learning are the most effective means of teaching students. I try to incorporate many different types of learning activities in hopes of holding the students' interest. I hope that students want to come to my rotation because the experiences are stimulating. I want learning to be exciting and fun. Education is a two-way process, and I expect the learners to come prepared and with a willingness to learn. I have accepted responsibility that I am there to help each student learn in the most effective way possible.

Assessment of both the teacher and the learners are critical in any teaching environment. I will employ the students' active teaching to other colleagues, students, and patients as a means to assess their progress. Rubrics will be provided so that the students have a clear understanding of my expectations. The value of teaching others is that the students will truly need to master the material to teach it. I will actively engage the learners in feedback sessions on a weekly basis to assess the effectiveness of both the site and the teacher in facilitating learning. I will use this feedback as a method to improve experiences for both the learners and the teacher.

My teaching philosophy is in its infancy. I will continue to use humor and passion to engage my learners and value feedback as a crucial part of the process. I hope to continue to grow as a teacher and reflect on how my teaching values are incorporated into my personal values.

most appropriate for helping the learner understand foundational skills and knowledge. It will be beneficial to all learners at some point in time, but it is primarily useful for students and residents in the beginning stages of their experiences. Keep in mind when assigning readings that there are limitations to this kind of activity. Textbooks can potentially become outdated and referral to primary literature is recommended in most instances. Verifying that the readings are at an appropriate depth for the learner will help them meet the rotation's learning objectives. You should also avoid assigning a reading without proper follow-up to discuss the assignments and ensure understanding of the material. Lectures should be used sparingly in the clinical curriculum. They can help the learner focus on the relevant facts but should not replace the learner's self-directed research. A way to enhance learning through lecturing is to use an interactive lecture technique such as asking well-developed questions throughout the lecture. By asking the learner to put the material into his or her own words to answer questions, the material can be reinforced.

Modeling is defined as providing an example for the learner to follow as the preceptor solves a patient care problem in real time. In this process, the learner is required to process information in a live setting to solve a clinical problem rather than reflect on decisions already made. This type of teaching is best used once the learner has established foundational knowledge and skills. Activities used in modeling include thinking out loud, sharing hunches, examining all sides of an issue, and providing a rationale for why each decision was made. In this way, the learner is given a basic format for solving a complex problem that can be used in many different clinical scenarios. Modeling can be very effective in residency training when the learner is just beginning to grasp the practical application of clinical knowledge. For this teaching encounter to be most successful, the preceptor should prepare the student for the encounter. Cluing the learner in to specific things to look for in the process of solving the problem is essential. For example, if you suspect a certain disease process is present, point out crucial labs that would signify the specific disease. Help the student begin to see what clues allowed you to come to your clinical conclusion. The preceptor should be prepared to explain the steps involved in the modeled behavior. This may be difficult for more seasoned preceptors who do things automatically. It may be beneficial for you to talk through the problem-solving process out loud before trying to model a certain behavior. After modeling a process, a discussion should follow including key take-home points to help foster the development of the learner.

Coaching occurs once a learner is ready to be an active member of a process. As a coach, the preceptor asks the learner to perform the skill that was previously modeled. The preceptor then provides feedback and direction so the learner can refine that skill. Depending on the task and the learner's stage, the preceptor may need to provide detailed instructions, reminders, or encouragement to guide the learner through the process. In this type of setting, the preceptor safely supervises while the learners are gaining hands-on experience. Immediate feedback is crucial to reinforce learning. In this case, as well as modeling, preceptors point out important cues for the learner to look for when approaching the scenario. Often, the preceptor will need to switch back and forth between modeling and coaching depending on the comfort level and skill level of the student.

Facilitation is a process that allows the learner to perform independently, while the preceptor remains available, if needed. In facilitating, the preceptor offers direct practice experiences to allow the learner to practice their decision-making skills. A debriefing of the activity occurs after the fact to review opportunities for improvement and recognize appropriate performance. Facilitation usually occurs when the preceptor has coached the learner and is confident in his or her ability to function independently, normally occurring toward the end of a learning experience. This process also involves self-evaluation, helping learners to be more independent and grow professionally. A good way to begin this process is to use self-evaluation in the scheduled feedback process. The more experienced learners, such as residents, should be encouraged to routinely engage in the process of self-evaluation. In most cases, newer students will need to be taught the skill of self-evaluation.

Self-evaluation is a difficult process and a little guidance can go a long way. First, have the students establish the criteria of a successful performance. Once this is completed, they should collect data on how they performed and compare it with the criteria for a successful performance. Help the students make a judgment of how they did and encourage them to decide how to improve the next performance. This change should be put into practice the next time the learner performs the task. The ability to evaluate one's own learning is a hallmark of a professional and necessary to cultivate lifelong learning.

Quick Tip

Facilitation should only occur when both the preceptor and the learner are confident in the learner's ability to function independently.

Because you will be teaching many students at different levels of learning, a preceptor must be proficient in each of the four roles. Introductory pharmacy practice experience (IPPE) students will require more direct instruction and modeling versus APPE students, who will benefit more from modeling and coaching. A residency preceptor should expect the resident to require significantly less direct instruction compared to APPE students and should be expected to make it to the facilitation process by the end of their residency.

CASE-BASED TEACHING

Case-based teaching allows the teacher to take the learner beyond the traditional lecture method of learning. This will aid learners in applying knowledge to direct patient care. Case-based teaching involves presenting the learner with a case to be solved. The focus may either be on a case that has been solved (during which the learner is walked through the steps of the process of solving the clinical scenario), or the learners may be given a case that requires their own problem solving skills to analyze the case and formulate a plan.

One of the biggest challenges in case-based teaching is helping the learner understand the thought process involved in clinical problem solving. Enough information should be provided to guide the students to understand why the preceptor made specific decisions without giving away the answers at first glance. This will help the learner develop clinical reasoning skills. Identifying errors or missed opportunities will also help learners refine their reasoning skills. You can also use directed questioning to guide students through the decision-making process.

As an alternative to traditional case-based presentations, the Five Minute Preceptor model has been advocated to maximize the effectiveness of learning.[3] This method encourages critical thinking, provides immediate feedback, and teaches in a time-efficient manner. It is meant to increase the quality and frequency of teaching in clinical settings where time constraints limit the amount of preceptor-student teaching encounters.

The Five Minute Preceptor model involves five steps:

♦ In *Step 1*, the student is required to take a stand. At this point in the process, the preceptor uses a general question to encourage the student to process information and provide some judgment about the clinical scenario. An example of a general question may be, "Tell me what is happening with your patient."

♦ At *Step 2*, the preceptor is probing for supporting evidence as to why the student came to the conclusion elicited in Step 1. An advanced learner may not need much probing but a beginning learner may need more substantial questioning. The preceptor's question may be, "What other information might you need to make this decision?" Through the probing process, the students' learning needs and knowledge gaps will become clear.

♦ *Step 3* allows the preceptor to teach general rules after the student takes a stand and defends his or her position. This step should include a maximum of three key points to ensure the learner retains the information. Providing too many take-home points usually causes the learner to forget a number of them and diminishes the effectiveness of the session.

The last two steps involve feedback.

♦ In *Step 4*, the preceptor should be reinforcing the positive aspects of the students' performance. The preceptor should comment on the appropriate knowledge, skills, and attitudes demonstrated so the student can apply these positives regularly.

♦ *Step 5* involves correcting any errors or misinterpretations. This should be done using constructive feedback intended to help the student improve future performance.

The Five Minute Preceptor model has been shown to be an efficient way to provide constructive feedback for both learner and teacher. By using open-ended questions, the preceptor stimulates discussion around the student's thought process. This type of teaching puts the focus on learners verbalizing their thought processes rather than passively following the preceptor's thought process. This also provides timely feedback to reinforce growth and learning.

Case Question

JK's APPE student is struggling to develop appropriate plans for the patients seen in clinic. Using the Five Minute Preceptor model, what are some questions that could be used by JK to help the student identify the primary problem and provide supporting evidence to back up his or her plans?

TEACHING CRITICAL THINKING SKILLS

Critical thinking is an important element for all healthcare disciplines to possess and is thought to be the hallmark of the effective practitioner. Critical thinking skills will allow the practitioner to respond appropriately to a wide variety of clinical situations by translating knowledge into practice.

Inductive and deductive reasoning are both involved in critical thinking. *Inductive reasoning* is the ability to consider all of the possibilities. This type of reasoning typically takes a considerable amount of time. *Deductive reasoning* is the weeding out of all possible solutions while obtaining data. New students may employ inductive reasoning because they do not have the ability to discriminate relevant from irrelevant data. A more advanced student or resident should be able to identify key data and determine the appropriate solution. Depending on the situation, the experienced practitioner is able to switch from one type of reasoning to another to solve a clinical problem. To teach the skills of critical thinking involves teaching the learner to discriminate the relevant from irrelevant, consider data from a variety of sources, organize data into a hypothesis, and to realize the repercussions of the hypothesis.

SOCRATIC METHOD

The Socratic method of teaching is a student-centered approach that challenges learners to develop their critical thinking skills and engage in discussion. In this method, the teacher questions students in a manner that requires them to consider how they rationalize and respond to certain topics. Ideally, the answers to questions are not a stopping point for thought but are, instead, a bridge to further analysis and research. The goal is to help students process information and engage in deeper understanding of topics. Asking the right questions is the prerequisite to critical thinking. Questions may have no single answer. They should be structured to create a dialogue that leads to a greater understanding of the topic, and require references to support the decision or hypothesis.[4]

Quick Tip

Silence can create a kind of helpful tension in pushing students to respond. Be willing to accept silence as productive.

OTHER METHODS

Additional teaching strategies can be employed to promote critical thinking. Essential to the teaching encounter is the knowledge, skill level, and the style of learning best suited to the learner. The teacher must take all factors into consideration when determining the best approach to teaching critical thinking skills.

The following are some strategies you might consider:

♦ The *thinking aloud* approach, as in modeling, occurs when the preceptor verbalizes the thought processes and the rationale of the actions while the situation is occurring. This verbalization of the thought process allows the learner to associate the process and the situation and gives a view to the preceptor's reasoning, thereby promoting understanding.

♦ *Debriefing* is a viable alternative. During debriefing the teacher and learner relive the experience shortly after it occurs with an explanation of the thoughts and actions.

♦ *Chart review* is another method that can be used to promote critical thinking. This can be done to help focus on the logical thought process as a preceptor reviews the chart with a student.

♦ *Simulated scenarios* can be used to enhance critical thinking skills as technology becomes more advanced. There are many advantages to using this type of scenario. The less skilled learner can work at his or her own pace and may be likely to participate if there is no negative consequence from an incorrect suggestion. It also provides a realistic experience for students to learn complex clinical skills in a safe environment without the threat of harming patients. Simulation makes it easier for preceptors to control the learning situation in contrast to the difficulty caused by time constraints and individual patient needs in clinical situations. Some examples of suggested scenarios include watching a practicing professional care for a patient and having the student identify good and bad performance aspects of the scenario. Other possible scenarios include suggesting how to handle patients in difficult situations or suggesting ways to handle anticipated problems if an incorrect decision is made.

A variety of strategies are effective in promoting and advancing critical thinking skills. The result can be the timely delivery of effective patient care in a complex clinical environment—skills a preceptor hopes a student will attain.

TEACHING EMOTIONAL INTELLIGENCE

Emotional intelligence is something in each of us that is a bit intangible, making it quite a challenge to teach. It can be described as a type of cognitive ability involving the ability to perceive, use, understand, and manage emotion. Thought to be a subset of social intelligence, emotional intelligence affects how we manage behavior, navigate social complexities, and make personal decisions to achieve positive results. Increasing research has shown that emotional intelligence influences one's ability to deliver safe and compassionate healthcare, making it a necessary part of any learning curriculum in a professional environment where every day work is emotionally charged.

Emotionally competent adults get along well with others. They communicate effectively, are cooperative, and learn to negotiate to solve problems. In other words, those who possess emotional intelligence "play nice in the sandbox." With the focus on the necessity of competently functioning interprofessional teams, wouldn't it be nice to have pharmacists who have learned to play nicely in this healthcare arena? Many of us realize that there are essential skills related to emotional intelligence, and you may be surprised to learn these skills can be taught to students. Emotional intelligence can be encompassed in a skill set that contains empathy, the ability to solve problems, optimism, and self-awareness. A person with a high level of emotional intelligence has the ability to join together emotions and reasoning, using emotions to facilitate such reasoning, and to reason intelligently about emotion.

There are five core emotional competencies that need to be developed in an individual who strives to be highly emotional intelligent. These include self-awareness, social awareness, self-management, relationship skills, and decision-making skills.[5] Refer to Table 5-1 for a detailed explanation of these competencies.

Table 5-1. Emotional Intelligence Competencies

Competency	Definition
Self-awareness	Knowing what we are feeling and having a realistic assessment of our own abilities and a well-grounded sense of self-confidence
Social awareness	The ability to consider others' perspectives and appreciate diversity while interacting with such groups in a positive manner
Self-management	The ability to control emotions so they facilitate rather than interfere with the objective
Relationship skills	Handling emotions in relationships effectively, displaying cooperation, and negotiating conflicts
Decision-making skills	Making decisions based on an accurate consideration of all relevant factors, the consequences of different courses of action, and taking responsibility for one's own actions

Source: Adapted from Collaborative for Academic, Social, and Emotional Learning (2003). Safe and Sound: An Educational Leader's Guide to Evidence-Based Social and Emotional Learning (SEL) Programs. Chicago, IL: CASEL.

Communication skills are related to developing emotional intelligence. Emotions become visible when linked to interactions with any type of verbal and nonverbal communication. Decisions about how, when, and what to say are related to the level of emotional intelligence. This type of skill can be measured through the evaluation of communication encounters between the student and either patients or colleagues. Giving feedback on communication skills will help students to conceptualize the how, when, and what of the process leading to self-awareness of their own emotional intelligence. As with any type of skill, the more interactions the learner has (and the more feedback given), the greater the competency in the skill. Providing students with opportunities to practice empathy, navigate conflict, and work within a team will help them build the competencies listed above and, in turn, develop emotional intelligence. When evaluating your learner's communication skills, it is important to have a set of competencies with which to evaluate them. Table 5-2 lists some recommendations to use when assessing communication skills.

If you have a student who is having difficulty with communication skills, you might try the following exercise. The objective of this exercise is to focus on listening without interpreting what another person is saying and to foster active listening skills. The preceptor chooses a topic to discuss in which there are both negative and positive sides. For example, this can be something simple, such as "I am having difficulty getting along with my roommate." The opposing approach is, "My roommate and I get along very well." One student gives the negative approach and the other student provides the positive approach. The students should face each other and share each of the following sentences one at a time without relating to the other person.

Table 5-2. Assessing Communication Skills

Questioning	Verbal Language	Nonverbal Language
Uses open-ended questions	Does not use complicated medical terminology	Squarely faces patient
Uses specific questions to help clarify information	Avoids slang	Maintains eye contact during most of the conversation
Avoids leading questions		Appropriate open posture

Student one: "I am having difficulty getting along with my roommate."

Student two: "My roommate and I get along very well."

Student one: "My roommate refuses to wash the dishes after she eats."

Student two: "My roommate and I each take turns doing the household chores."

Student one: "My roommate likes to have loud parties every Saturday at our apartment."

Student two: "My roommate and I often hang out on weekends and either study or watch movies."

At this point, a discussion should occur that encompasses the following questions: Can you think of times when you are trying to listen to another person while your own thoughts are racing? What was it like to share without your partner responding to what you said? You can use the answers to these questions as a springboard to discuss previous interactions with patients. Ask the students if there are times they have not been listening to the patient but, instead, were focused on their next question. Ask how it felt to share and have no judgment in a response. Did it feel safe and more comfortable to share if you knew the next statement would be nonjudgmental?

Next, the students will practice reflection. In this exercise, each student shares his or her opinion (one sentence at a time), and the other student responds by paraphrasing. Each student takes turns paraphrasing what the other student says. After the exercise goes a few rounds, discuss the following questions: What was it like to paraphrase what your partner said? What gets in the way of representing what the other person was saying? Were you aware of your own bias, judgments, or perceptions interfering with simply restating their point? Reflection is a very powerful tool in communication and sends the message to the other party that you are listening and also will allow for correction of any misunderstood communication.

Successful teamwork is essential in today's healthcare system. This means that emotional intelligence, in the form of empathy and collaboration, is more important than ever. A team-building exercise can help your students perfect these skills and increase emotional intelligence. To begin, ask your students to focus on the team they are rounding with and provide four examples of different skills that each member of the team may portray. These can include *acting* (gets things done), *speculating* (looks at the big picture before acting), *caring* (considers feelings before acting), and *detailing* (pays attention to small details). Have the students identify where they best fit within these descriptions and where each teammate fits. It is perfectly acceptable to come up with your own descriptors, as well, if they would better describe your team. Next, lead a discussion on the value of the different styles and the positive and negative attributes of each. Discuss how knowing each other's style allows the team to work more effectively. This activity increases awareness of the student's own style, as well as the styles of other teammates, opening the door to empathy and an appreciation of diversity.

ASSESSING EMOTIONAL INTELLIGENCE

To assess emotional intelligence in the learner, focus on your student's self-directed skills, such as awareness of their own emotions, control of impulses, and regulation of their emotions. Focus on how the student makes empathetic statements, elicits patient concerns, and communicates emotions to others. The crux of the assessment should assess the student's awareness and management of the patient's emotions along with his or her own. Giving feedback in each of the student's encounters is critical for him or her to start to develop self-awareness and understanding of how he or she makes decisions related to navigating emotions. You may also consider assigning a written reflection of the situation.

The reflection should answer the following questions:

◆ What did the patient/colleague say?
◆ What did the student say or what was he or she thinking?
◆ What should the student have said or how could he or she have improved the interaction?

Reflection is a very valuable tool to help develop a learner's self-awareness. Requiring the learner to reflect on how he or she could have done it better gives the learner a valuable map to follow in future interactions.

> ### *Case Question*
>
> *MJ is a preceptor at a very busy retail pharmacy. She has assigned her APPE student to ring out prescriptions and counsel each patient about the medication he or she is receiving. You overhear a very disgruntled patient questioning the student as to why the prescription is taking so long. After the third inquiry, the student's tone of voice changes to that of annoyance. When the prescription is ready for pick-up, you note the student fails to offer counseling. How could MJ use the reflection process to help the student navigate negative emotions when dealing with disgruntled customers?*

Healthcare is an emotionally demanding practice and emotions clearly influence how health professionals identify, perceive, interpret, and act on information. Always consider how a learner's culture may influence his or her interpretation, display, and discourse related to emotions. While you are assessing the emotional intelligence of

Table 5-3. Sample Critical Thinking and Emotional Intelligence Activities

Critical Thinking Activities	Emotional Intelligence Activities
Create a drug diary detailing an in-depth exploration of a group of medications to treat a condition. Review the pathophysiology of the disease, presenting symptoms, and the clinical rationale for how the drugs correct the pathophysiology and symptoms.	Have the student reflect on an emotional response a difficult patient is having and discuss how to best handle the conflict.
Create a concept map for a disease, a class of drugs, or a medication-use process. A concept map is a tool that illustrates relationships between concepts usually presented by graphing these concepts in a hierarchical fashion.	Keep a journal and document the emotional situations you experience each day. Review these scenarios with your students each week.
Explain to a patient how a drug works. How would this differ if you were explaining it to a physician? Why and what assumptions did you make when you were developing each explanation?	Ask students to debate a scenario related to medical ethics.

your learner, you must be emotionally competent, as well. Be fully aware of your own emotions and the effect of your behavior on the students. There are a number of emotional intelligence assessments available online (see Suggested Reading). Table 5-3 lists additional sample activities to promote emotional intelligence and stimulate critical thinking.

THE GIST

1. Periodically reflect on your teaching philosophy to promote your growth as both a teacher and a healthcare professional.
2. There are four different roles a preceptor can assume (direct instruction, modeling, coaching, and facilitating). Assess the learning needs of each student before deciding which role you should assume.
3. Critical thinking is a necessary component of the decision-making process and a skill that every practicing professional should possess.
4. Healthcare is an emotionally demanding practice that necessitates a high level of emotional intelligence to navigate the aspects of patient care and teamwork. Teaching and assessing emotional intelligence is a key responsibility for preceptors.

SUGGESTED READING

MindTools. https://www.mindtools.com/pages/article/ei-quiz.htm (accessed 6 April 2016). This site provides an emotional intelligence self-assessment quiz.

Savoy M, Yunyongying P. Can a simplified approach to emotional intelligence be the key to learner-centered teaching? *J Grad Med Educ*. 2014; 211-4.

REFERENCES

1. Kearns K, Sullivan CS. Resources and practices to help graduate students and postdoctoral fellows write statements of teaching philosophy. *Adv Physiol Educ*. 2011; 35:136-45.

2. Weitzel KW, Walters EA, Taylor J. Teaching clinical problem solving: a preceptor's guide. *Am J Health-Syst Pharm*. 2012; 69:1588-99.

3. Bott G, Mohide EA, Lawlor Y. Clinical teaching technique for nurse preceptors: the five minute preceptor. *Prof Nurs*. 2011; 27:35-42.

4. Ross V. The Socratic method: what it is and how to use it in the classroom. *Speak Teach*. 2003;13(1):1-4.

5. Collaborative for Academic, Social and Emotional Learning. Safe and sound: an educational leader's guide to Evidence-Based Social and Emotional Learning (SEL) Program. 2003. http://indiana.edu/~pbisin/pdf/Safe_and_Sound.pdf.

Chapter 6

Assessing Learner Performance

S. Scott Wisneski

CASE STUDY

BK is a clinical pharmacist at a community teaching hospital currently precepting TT, who is completing a 4-week acute care advanced pharmacy practice experience (APPE). Since starting, TT has been late to the rotation on three separate occasions and is having difficulty answering drug-related questions. BK is concerned about TT's performance and feels this student needs to receive some formal feedback before things get worse. Since BK is a fairly new preceptor, she seeks advice from her colleagues in the department on how best to provide feedback to TT. She is considering waiting until the scheduled midpoint evaluation later next week to express her concerns to TT.

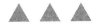

INTRODUCTION

Assessment of a student or resident's skills is an essential component of experiential training. An effective preceptor must carefully and honestly evaluate learners to ensure they have developed the skills necessary to be successful pharmacists. Assessing learners can be challenging for a preceptor who may find the process uncomfortable or believes it will negatively impact their relationship. If an adequate assessment is not performed, learners will be at a significant disadvantage with regard to their professional and personal development. In cases where self-evaluation skills are poor (a common weakness for trainees), the learners may even believe all is going well when the opposite is actually the case. A quality evaluation that is delayed until the end of a rotation leaves the learner with no opportunity to make improvements to his or her performance. This chapter will provide you with techniques in giving effective formative feedback and a summative midpoint evaluation to your students or residents.

ASSESSMENT VERSUS FEEDBACK

Assessment is either *formative* or *summative*.[1] Formative assessment, commonly referred to as *feedback*, is an ongoing evaluation of the learner during the experience focused on reinforcing, developing, or correcting specific behaviors. Summative assessment, on the other hand, is a measure of one's global achievement during the experience with the purpose of providing a grade. Characteristics of formative and summative assessments are provided in Table 6-1.

WHY PROVIDE FEEDBACK?

Providing effective feedback is imperative to help the learner reach his or her maximum potential during the experience. Feedback reinforces good practice, corrects mistakes, and modifies the learner's behavior in the future. When done effectively, feedback can raise the learner's self-awareness and leave him or her with the information required to hone their future actions. Providing praise for good performance can have a motivating

Table 6-1. Elements of Formative and Summative Assessments

	Formative Assessment	Summative Assessment
Timing	Shortly after completing an activity or skill	Scheduled at the midpoint and end of the experience
Setting	Informal, short discussion	Formal, extended discussion
Scope	Focused on specific actions or behaviors, nonjudgmental	Global performance, provides a definitive assessment
Purpose	Reinforces good practice, corrects mistakes, and modifies behavior. Allows the student to continue to reach the goals of the experience.	Grading the experience, providing suggestions for future experiences. Examines how the student performed in meeting the goals of the experience.

effect on the learner to continue acting in a positive way. On the other hand, corrective feedback enables the learners to recognize the outcome of their actions and urges them to alter their behavior to achieve a more desirable result. Reasons for providing feedback are listed in Box 6-1.

BOX 6-1. PROVIDING FEEDBACK WILL:

- Develop learner's ability to perform operational, clinical, and professional skills
- Increase learner's confidence
- Improve the learning process for the learner
- Encourage the learner to try new skills
- Improve overall performance of the learner
- Reinforce good behaviors
- Identify areas of needed improvement
- Foster continuous professional development
- Emphasize the preceptor's expectations
- Allow the learner to provide a self-assessment

Although recognized as being essential for learning, learners often report receiving little feedback.[2] When formative assessments are completed, they are often too late, lack detail, or have limited utility. Learners have identified the ability to give feedback as one of the most important qualities of a good preceptor, second only to clinical competence.[2] Even though informal assessment is seen as a crucial skill by learners, there are numerous reasons preceptors may not give feedback to their learners (see Box 6-2).

BOX 6-2. YOUR REASONS FOR NOT PROVIDING FEEDBACK MAY BE:

- You are uncomfortable with calling attention to negative behavior
- You fear you may adversely affect a learner's self-esteem or the teacher-student relationship
- You lack the time to give feedback
- The lack of acceptance of your feedback by previous learners
- You fear you may do more harm than good by being too critical
- The learner may be defensive
- A behavior appears to be a one-time occurrence not warranting feedback
- Your learners do not recognize when feedback is being given
- You lack training regarding learner skill level or development expectations

---

Feedback is a crucial part of a learner's maturation. When feedback is not provided, a learner's good performance is not reinforced and, more critically, poor performance will likely remain uncorrected. The learner may then rely on hearsay from other staff or colleagues to gain the desired feedback. The learner may even self-determine his or her level of competence and resort to learning through trial and error. When the end of the experience arrives, the learner is left unsure of his or her progress and unable to make a plan for future development.

PROVIDING EFFECTIVE FEEDBACK

Starting on the first day of the rotation, you should discuss how feedback will be provided to your learner. During this early discussion, the preceptor should emphasize the purpose of feedback, how it will be delivered, and when it will be given. Ideally, the preceptor should strive to give feedback following completion of essential activities that the student is expected to demonstrate competence in performing. Do not wait until the end of the experience to provide feedback. In a busy practice, you may consider taking some time at the beginning or end of the day to provide feedback to the learners. Some may use the end of each week as an opportunity to provide a student or resident with a more detailed feedback session. This is a good opportunity to identify other activities or competencies the learner will work on during the coming week.

The following are key principles you can use when providing effective feedback to your learners:

- *Label your discussion as feedback*—As mentioned earlier, learners often report that they do not get enough feedback from their preceptors. In some cases, they may not recognize the information provided by their preceptor as feedback. You should label the discussion or what you are about to say as "feedback." For example, start the discussion with a statement such as, "I would like to offer you some feedback on your performance on morning rounds today."

- *Provide feedback in private*—When providing feedback, it should be done in a private, relaxed setting free from distraction. The discussion should not be done where it can be observed by patients, staff, and other learners. Make sure you respect the privacy of your learner to avoid any potential embarrassment.

- *Feedback should be timely, regular, and frequent*—The closer to the activity you provide feedback, the better it will be for the learner. Identifying the essential performance-related activities beforehand can help determine when feedback will be given. Close proximity to the activity also helps to easily recognize the specific skills to reinforce and those needing further development. Giving feedback regularly limits the potential for poor performance to get out of hand and allows time to correct behavior. Feedback should not be a one-time event or only occur when something negative happens.

- *Feedback should be specific and descriptive*—The preceptor should avoid statements such as, "You are doing fine," "Very good performance," or "You are not meeting the objectives." Statements like these do not include specific details justifying such comments. Tying specific details of the student's performance to your feedback is key to allowing the student to develop self-assessment skills. For example, if the student is not meeting your expectations with regard to professionalism, indicate the specific traits or behaviors that caused him or her to fall below the bar.

♦ *Feedback should focus on behaviors, not personal traits*—Emphasize specific behaviors that can be reinforced or improved. Focus on what was observed about the learner's performance. For example, instead of saying "Your tardiness is unacceptable and will no longer be tolerated," try "I noticed you have been late for rotation the last 3 days." The learner can then focus on the specific behavior that needs to be improved.

♦ *Limit the amount of information*—Try not to overwhelm your student during feedback sessions by discussing too many behaviors. Focus on no more than two to three issues in each session. Otherwise, your learner may feel attacked, demoralized, or may not be able to retain all of the feedback delivered. Prioritize the most important feedback that needs to be given immediately and make note of the less important issues that could be brought up at a later time.

♦ *Talk to others about the learner's performance*—Consult your pharmacist colleagues, technicians, and other site staff to obtain their observations of your learner's performance. When students participate on interprofessional teams, it creates an excellent opportunity to seek feedback from other team members. This can provide a more complete picture of the learner's overall performance.

♦ *Provide specific steps to correct shortcomings*—The preceptor and learner should agree on what needs to be done to improve performance. Set specific, measurable goals or plans for future performance.

♦ *Remember that the purpose of feedback is to improve performance*—When feedback is provided, make an effort to check in on your learner's progress on the established plan. It may be beneficial to keep a few notes from informal feedback sessions to make it easier to track your student's development.

♦ *Use one of the common approaches to providing feedback*—Use the approaches discussed in the next section to lend structure to your feedback sessions.

Quick Tip

No preceptor perfectly executes all of the elements of effective feedback. Asking your trainees to provide feedback on your feedback is a great way to gain an outside perspective on your assessment style. Waiting until after grades are submitted helps ensure honest feedback is provided.

APPROACHES TO PROVIDING FEEDBACK

There are a number of approaches to effectively providing feedback. No one method is better than another, so consider trying out a number of styles to see which suits you best.

♦ *Feedback sandwich*—This commonly used approach starts with providing a positive statement followed by a corrective statement and then closes with another reinforcing statement.[3] Thus, the corrective feedback is "sandwiched" between the two reinforcing feedback statements. For example:

 ■ *Reinforcing feedback*—*"You are well-prepared for medical team rounds. Your level of preparation allows you to be an active participant on the team by providing an accurate and current list of the patients' medication-related problems."*

- *Corrective feedback*—"I have also noticed that you have been 15 minutes late for the start of rounds the last 3 days. The attending physician noticed your late arrival and pulled me aside to discuss it."
- *Reinforcing feedback*—"The information you provided the team on the patient's antibiotic therapy was evidenced-based and well presented. Members of the team had some key questions that you were able to answer with accuracy."

A benefit of this technique is that it softens the impact of the criticism or corrective feedback for the learner. This can make it easier for your learner to accept the negative feedback and avoid defensive posturing. Preceptors who are uncomfortable with providing negative comments find the feedback sandwich easier than simply focusing on negative feedback, although some preceptors may feel that the key corrective feedback may appear to be watered-down. A common mistake in using the feedback sandwich is using the word "but" before giving the corrective feedback. In doing so, a learner may quickly ignore the reinforcing statements and focus on what is said after the "but." You can overcome this habit by just stating the corrective feedback. A suggested modification a preceptor may want to consider to the feedback sandwich is replacing the closing praise statement with outlining a plan for improving the corrective feedback. This simple alteration helps to identify and discuss the actions your learner can take to improve his or her performance moving forward.

- *Pendleton Four-Step Model*—This method allows the learner to provide his or her own comments on what was positive with the performance and what areas are in need of improvement.[4] This is followed by the preceptor's validation of the learner's comments and further elaboration on performance. The four steps of this model are as follows:
  - *Step 1:* The learner is asked to state what is good about his or her performance.
  - *Step 2:* The preceptor states areas of agreement and elaborates on good performance.
  - *Step 3:* The learner is asked to describe the areas of performance that could be improved.
  - *Step 4:* The preceptor states what he or she has observed that could be improved.

Compared with the feedback sandwich, the Pendleton Model lends itself to a two-way discussion between learner and preceptor. By encouraging self-assessment, learners develop self-awareness of their own strengths and weaknesses. Including a specific improvement plan as part of the fourth step will add to the overall effectiveness of this technique. The step-wise structure of this method may cause the preceptor to refrain from addressing additional problems that do not come out in the learner's own assessment. It is important to address other concerns you have with the learner as part of the discussion.

- *Situation-Behavior-Impact (SBI) Feedback Tool*— Developed by the Center for Creative Leadership, the SBI Feedback Tool includes three distinct parts: situation, behavior, and impact.[5]
  - *Situation*—First, the preceptor defines the when and where of the performance to be addressed. This helps to put the feedback into context and gives the learner a specific setting and time of reference. For example:

- "During yesterday morning's team rounds, when you were answering the resident's drug information question regarding warfarin . . ."

- *Behavior*—The second step allows the preceptor to describe the specific behaviors that need to be addressed. It is important that only those behaviors you actually witnessed are discussed. Do not make assumptions or provide subjective judgment about those behaviors. For example, if you observe the student providing incorrect information to the resident's inquiry about warfarin, do not assume the student did not prepare thoroughly. Simply comment on the actual error made. Use measurable information to describe the behavior, ensuring the feedback remains objective.

- *Impact*—Finally, the preceptor describes how the behavior affected the student or others. If applicable, consider including the impact the behavior would have on a patient. For example:

  - "During yesterday morning's rounds, when you were answering the resident's drug information question on warfarin you made a mistake regarding the effect of an interaction between warfarin, erythromycin, and amiodarone. This could potentially have had a serious impact on the patient if the resident prescribed these drugs together."

The preceptor should encourage the learner to reflect further about the performance, recognize the impact of his or her behavior, and consider specific actions to prevent a similar problem in the future. Although this example utilized the SBI method to deliver negative feedback, this model can be used to provide positive feedback, as well. In this situation, the impact on the preceptor or patient would be positive. This encourages the learner to recognize his or her effect on others. You may provide suggestions to achieve an even greater impact in the future.

Case Question

BK is nervous to confront her student regarding her tardiness. Choose one of the frameworks for effective feedback and describe how it can be used to lend structure to the session and lessen the anxiety BK is feeling.

Even for preceptors comfortable with the principles and techniques outlined above, it can still be difficult to incorporate regular feedback into the day-to-day hustle and bustle of the practice site. A suggestion is to identify specific activities the learner will perform during the rotation as triggers to giving feedback.

Examples of activities that should trigger feedback include:

- A formal presentation (e.g., patient case, journal club)
- Answering a drug information question
- A patient counseling session
- Making a recommendation during rounds
- Completion of a project
- Completion of a practice skill performed for the first time (e.g., transfer of a prescription, giving an immunization, preparing a sterile product)

These activities are ideal times to give your learner some feedback. You will find that learners want and expect that you will be giving some form of assessment following these types of activities.

To assist preceptors in giving activity-related feedback, colleges of pharmacy often have assessment tools or rubrics that can be used to assess learner performance. Examples of assessment tools from one college of pharmacy are provided in Appendixes 6A through 6C.

Your institution or pharmacy may have similar tools you can use, while some preceptors find it beneficial to create their own tool. An added advantage of using one of these assessment tools is that it can provide talking points you can use as part of the feedback session. This helps to keep the feedback focused on specific behaviors or skills. Finally, an assessment rubric also provides documented assessment of the learner's performance. These documents may be helpful to support later summative evaluations.

Quick Tip

Using the same rubric over the course of a learning experience will give you the chance to track your trainee's progression. Because the document is standardized, there is a smaller chance that biases or grade inflation will skew your assessment.

GIVING DIFFICULT FEEDBACK

Giving difficult or negative feedback to a learner can be challenging, even for the experienced preceptor. The effective preceptor can overcome initial hesitancy to provide this type of feedback utilizing the five steps outlined below.[6]

1. *Reframe bad news*—When administering feedback to a learner who is not meeting expectations, there is the tendency to conclude it is bad news. Although, in reality, you are being honest with the intent of helping the learner become a successful pharmacist. The preceptor should frame the news in such a way to put the emphasis on it as constructive criticism so the learner will be able to achieve a high level of success in the future. Even though the student or resident may not like what is being said, he or she will develop an appreciation for the preceptor when bad news is being discussed in this manner.

2. *Come out with it*—A common tendency when giving difficult feedback is to not directly come out with it to the learner. Do not dance around the issue or stammer through the exchange because the learner may pick up on your hesitancy to deliver the bad news. The effective preceptor should state the issue directly. Present the issue in a respectful manner, focusing on the behavior itself and not the learner's personal traits.

3. *Be specific and actionable*—As discussed above, negative feedback should be specific and contain a stepwise plan to improve the student's poor performance. If the preceptor's expectations are unclear, the learner may not know what or how

to correct poor performance. Make sure your learner understands the concern and has an agreed-on plan to move forward toward success.

4. *Listen and coach*—There can be a tendency for preceptors to dominate the discussion to the point where the learner is not engaged in resolving the issue, especially if the preceptor is upset or angry. You should allow time for learners to provide their own thoughts about what they are hearing. Taking the time to listen can help preceptors identify the thought process that led to poor results. If you are feeling angry or upset about the situation, it may be a good idea to refrain from discussing it with the learner until you have some time to cool off. Tell the learner how you are presently feeling, that you need to take some time to think more about the issue, and that you will discuss it at a future day and time.

5. *Remember to praise*—You should also point out what is working well along with what needs additional work. Indicate the areas where performance is meeting or exceeding expectations. This can help to build up and motivate the learner to perform better in the future rather than leaving him or her feeling like a failure and incapable of demonstrating a high level of achievement. Keep in mind not to give unjustified praise that could potentially dilute or minimize the behaviors in need of a change.

Although it is often unpleasant to give students or residents difficult feedback, using these points will increase your skill and confidence as these situations present themselves. The key thing is that you remain calm, professional, and display a sense of caring for your learner.

The following are examples of situations when negative feedback should obviously be provided to the learner:

♦ Displaying unprofessional behavior
♦ Not being prepared for the rotation activities
♦ Not completing an assignment
♦ Committing an error that potentially could result in a negative effect on a patient or the practice site
♦ Not demonstrating behavior focused on continuous professional development

When these types of behaviors surface, it is important to document each occurrence thoroughly and seek the guidance of the director of experiential education or residency program director as soon as possible.

Quick Tip

Consider having someone else (e.g., residency director, director of pharmacy, fellow preceptor) present when you give negative feedback to a learner.

> ## Case Question
>
> *BK is beginning to feel that TT's poor performance stems from his lack of interest in her practice area. Why would these feelings be inappropriate to include in a feedback session for TT's performance on rounds?*

GIVING A MIDPOINT EVALUATION

Generally, half way through a rotation is an excellent time to consider administering a midpoint evaluation. In contrast to the formative feedback you give throughout the rotation, midpoint evaluations are summative in nature. These evaluations are an ideal time for you and the learner to meet and globally assess performance. The midpoint summarizes what has occurred and reinforces the preceptor's expectations. In some cases, this evaluation will include an actual grade the learner has earned. The learner should have a clear idea of how he or she is performing and what needs to occur over the remaining portion of the rotation. Completing a midpoint evaluation ensures that all parties are aware of the learner's progress to date, limiting the chance for surprises at the end of the experience.

The following are key parameters in preparing and giving a midpoint evaluation:

♦ *Review requirements for midpoint evaluations*—As part of preparing for a student or resident rotation, you should review any requirements from the school of pharmacy or residency program regarding midpoint evaluations. Recently released standards from the Accreditation Council for Pharmacy Education (ACPE) indicate that, at a minimum, performance competence be documented midway through an APPE rotation and at its completion.[7] For residencies, ASHP does not require midpoint evaluations, but they would be highly recommended when a resident is not meeting expectations. Some programs may require midpoints for early rotations but back off from them as the resident demonstrates proficiency over the course of the year. The evaluation forms and grading process should be reviewed so there is a clear understanding of what is expected at the midpoint.

♦ *Discuss your plan for the midpoint evaluation with the learner*—Early in the rotation (preferably at orientation), the preceptor should discuss how a midpoint evaluation will be used. You may also select a specific date for the evaluation so that all parties are on the same page.

♦ *Prepare the evaluation*—In preparing the midpoint, you should be providing an assessment of the learner's global performance and progress to date. Unlike formative feedback that focuses on a single skill, midpoint evaluations should review the learner's proficiency in all of the assigned objectives. Including specific examples can be helpful so the learner has a clear understanding of their performance. Vague comments such as, "The student is doing fine" or "The resident's performance on rounds needs improvement" do little to help a learner. If possible, the midpoint should include a grade for the student's performance. This grade can provide an indication if the student or resident is passing or not passing at the present time. A specific plan of activities for the remaining portion of the rotation should be included in the midpoint, as well. If the learner is not meeting the preceptor's expectations, the midpoint should provide a plan for improvement. The improvement plan should be specific and include the expectations for successful completion. In some cases, the preceptor may want to discuss this plan with the student's experiential director or the resident's program director. This helps to inform administrators that the learner is not meeting the preceptor's expectations and that a plan is in place to get them on the right track.

♦ *Administering the evaluation*—The preceptor should formally review the midpoint with their learner. This should occur in private, encouraging a two-way discussion between the preceptor and learner. Because self-assessment is such a crucial part of the evaluation process, you may choose to kick off the midpoint with the learner describing their own performance. The preceptor should then provide his or her evaluation of the performance. Areas of improvement should be presented, including the specific behaviors that need to be changed. The plan for the remaining portion of the rotation should then be discussed. This is a great opportunity to reinforce your expectations of the learner for the remainder of the rotation. Any plan for improvement should be thoroughly discussed with the learner to ensure understanding and acceptance of the plan.

♦ *Post evaluation*—Following administration of the midpoint evaluation, the preceptor should ensure the learner's experiential director or resident's director receives a copy. As the rotation proceeds from this point onward, you should continue to provide formative feedback to the learner. In some situations, it may be appropriate for the preceptor to complete another formal summative evaluation of the learner's performance at some point before the final evaluation (especially if there were grave concerns about the learner's performance in the first half of the rotation). This can be done as a method to formally track the progress of the learner who may have significant issues with performance. This also provides additional documentation of the communication of expectations and poor performance should he or she not pass the rotation experience.

Quick Tip

Determine the requirements for administering a midpoint evaluation to your students or residents. Including this information in your syllabus will keep your learners informed of the assessment plan.

Case Question

Should BK wait until the midpoint to provide feedback to TT? What should she include in her midpoint evaluation of TT?

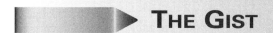

THE GIST

1. Providing effective formative feedback and summative assessment to students and residents is essential to the development and assessment of skills.
2. Characteristics of effective feedback include administering it in a private setting, being timely and frequent, specifically focusing on behaviors, and including a plan for improvement and follow-up.
3. Using various approaches, such as the feedback sandwich or others, can be effective ways of presenting feedback to the learner.
4. Giving difficult or negative feedback can be challenging but you can overcome the barriers through reframing, being direct, remaining specific to the concern, allowing the learner to self-assess, and coaching the learner to better performance.
5. Providing a midpoint evaluation is a formal way of providing your learner with an assessment of his or her performance and provides formal guidance for the remaining portion of the experience.

REFERENCES

1. King J. Giving feedback. *BMJ*. 1999; 318:S2-7200.
2. Bienstock JL, Katz NT, Cox SM et al. To the point: medical education reviews—providing feedback. *Am J Obstet Gynecol*. 2007; 196:508-13.
3. Cantillon P, Sargeant J. Teaching rounds: giving feedback in clinical settings. *BMJ*. 2008; 337:1292-4.
4. Pendleton D, Schofield T, Tate P et al. *The Consultation: An Approach to Learning and Teaching*. New York: Oxford University Press; 2003.
5. Center for Creative Leadership. SBI feedback process. https://www.ccl.org/leadership/pdf/community/SBIFeedbackProcess.pdf. Accessed 1 Dec 2015.
6. TrainManagers.com. Giving difficult feedback: 5 steps to telling inconvenient truths. http://www.trainmanagers.com/giving-difficult-feedback-5-steps-to-telling-inconvenient-truths/. Accessed 1 Dec 2015.
7. Accreditation Council for Pharmacy Education. Accreditation standards and key elements for the professional program in pharmacy leading to the doctor of pharmacy degree. 2015. https://www.acpe-accredit.org/pdf/Standards2016FINAL.pdf. Accessed 29 Feb 2016.

◆ APPENDIX 6A ◆

Evaluation of Journal Club

Student Name:_____ Evaluator:_____ Date:_____

MC = meets competency, NI = needs improvement, O = omitted

MC	NI	O	Criteria	Comments: Strengths and Areas for Improvement
☐ ☐ ☐ ☐ ☐	☐ ☐ ☐ ☐ ☐	☐ ☐ ☐ ☐ ☐	BACKGROUND ◆ States the title, journal of publication, and author affiliations (if relevant) ◆ Background information from the article was succinctly presented ◆ Other literature (e.g., previous articles, guidelines, etc.) was discussed in context of the article being presented ◆ The study objective(s) was/were clearly stated ◆ The study's sponsor and his or her role are identified (if applicable)	
☐ ☐ ☐ ☐ ☐ ☐ ☐	☐ ☐ ☐ ☐ ☐ ☐ ☐	☐ ☐ ☐ ☐ ☐ ☐ ☐	METHODS ◆ The study design (e.g., randomized controlled, cohort, case-control, etc.) was clearly and concisely described ◆ The study intervention was clearly and concisely described ◆ The study population was characterized ◆ Relevant inclusion/exclusion criteria were presented ◆ The primary (and secondary where applicable) endpoints were presented ◆ An accurate summary of the statistics was given ◆ Appropriateness (or lack thereof) of the statistical tests used was vocalized by the presenter	
☐ ☐ ☐ ☐	☐ ☐ ☐ ☐	☐ ☐ ☐ ☐	RESULTS ◆ Baseline characteristics of the study population were discussed ◆ The primary (and secondary, where applicable) results were presented ◆ The statistical significance (or lack thereof) of the results was noted ◆ The clinical significance (or lack thereof) of the results was noted	

Source: Courtesy of Northeast Ohio Medical University College of Pharmacy, Rootstown, OH.

MC	NI	O	Criteria	Comments: Strengths and Areas for Improvement
☐	☐	☐	CONCLUSIONS ♦ The author(s) conclusion(s) were presented	
☐	☐	☐	♦ Strengths and limitations as noted by the authors were presented	
☐	☐	☐	♦ Strengths and limitations identified by the student (aside from the authors) were presented	
☐	☐	☐	♦ The students conclusion(s) were presented	
☐	☐	☐	♦ Impact on clinical practice was presented	

MC	NI	Criteria	Comments: Strengths and Areas for Improvement
☐	☐	ABILITY TO ANSWER QUESTIONS ♦ Answered questions logically and accurately. If unsure of answer, the student clearly stated so	
☐	☐	♦ Responded to >50% of questions without assistance from instructor or other participants	
☐	☐	OVERALL PRESENTATION/DELIVERY ♦ Presentation was generally in a logical sequence	
☐	☐	♦ Presentation was within the allotted time	
☐	☐	♦ Spoke audibly to the audience	
☐	☐	♦ Used few (or no) distracters (e.g., "um") or distracting mannerisms (e.g., clicking pen)	
☐	☐	♦ Referred to notes occasionally but did not read from notes	
☐	☐	HANDOUT ♦ Handout was well organized, clear, and succinct	
☐	☐	♦ Appropriate references were cited in the proper format	

Pass or fail (circle one)

(Passing = ≥70% of MCs for applicable items)

Professional conduct (failure to achieve in this area will result in a meeting with the course director):
The student was:
☐ Dressed appropriately
☐ Wearing a clean white coat
☐ Displaying a name badge
☐ Respectful to other presenters

♦ **APPENDIX 6B** ♦

Case Presentation Evaluation

Resident/Student Name: _____ Topic: _____ Date: _____
MC = meets competency, NI = needs improvement

Patient presentation: demographic data, HPI, other history			
MC	**NI**	**Criteria**	**Comments**
☐	☐	♦ Opening statement provided patient identifier (initials), age, gender, race, and chief complaint	
☐	☐	♦ CC is stated in patient's own words	
☐	☐	♦ HPI was generally complete (including symptom analysis, historical context of problem, related medical history items)	
☐	☐	♦ PMH included and complete	
☐	☐	♦ FH/SH included and complete	
☐	☐	♦ Patient's medication history and allergies reported	
☐	☐	♦ Pertinent ROS findings included	

Patient presentation: lab/diagnostic data, physical exam findings			
MC	**NI**	**Criteria**	**Comments**
☐	☐	♦ Labs and diagnostic data findings required to assess the problem(s) reports OR if data unavailable, reported lab and diagnostic data that would be needed for full assessment	
☐	☐	♦ Vital signs reported	
☐	☐	♦ Physical exam data required to assess the problem(s) reported	

Patient presentation: assessment			
MC	**NI**	**Criteria**	**Comments**
☐	☐	♦ Assessment complete, includes primary problem, severity of primary problem, evidence to support this finding, likely cause of primary problem and current therapy	
☐	☐	♦ Problems appropriately prioritized from most severe to least severe	

Source: Courtesy of Northeast Ohio Medical University College of Pharmacy, Rootstown, OH.

Disease state discussion			
MC	**NI**	**Criteria**	**Comments**
☐	☐	◆ Provides a concise summary of epidemiology, etiology, pathophysiology and risk factors	
☐	☐	◆ Discusses patient presentation and pertinent diagnostic	
☐	☐	criteria	
		◆ Discusses all relevant pharmacological and	
☐	☐	nonpharmacological treatment options	
		◆ Includes brief discussion of evidence-based guidelines and	
☐	☐	primary literature for treating disease state being discussed	
		◆ Lists goals/endpoints of therapy and timeframes associated	
☐	☐	with meeting goals/endpoints	
		◆ Lists appropriate follow-up and monitoring of disease state	

Treatment plan and critique of care			
MC	**NI**	**Criteria**	**Comments**
☐	☐	◆ States a specific drug therapy recommendation (generic name, dose, route of administration, dosing frequency, and duration)	
☐	☐	◆ States patient-specific considerations present in case that impact choice of the drugs and/or drug classes being considered for the primary problem (at a minimum)	
☐	☐	◆ Accurately states agent-related variables, including information about comparative efficacy, safety, cost, and convenience of the drugs and/or drug classes being considered for the primary problem (at a minimum)	
☐	☐	◆ Lists specific measurable parameters (subjective and objective) that enable the practitioner to assess for efficacy and toxicity of the recommendation	
☐	☐	◆ Includes frequency of monitoring for each parameter that is consistent with standards of care, and/or the severity of the problem	
☐	☐	◆ Accurately identifies drug-related problems with patient's home medication regimen	
☐	☐	◆ Includes critique of treatment of the primary problem (at a minimum)	

Additional comments:

Pass/fail (circle one)

Evaluator name:_____

CC = chief complaint; HPI = history of present illness; FH/SH = family history/social history; PMH = past
medical history; ROS = review of systems.

◆ APPENDIX 6C ◆

Verbal Patient Counseling Rubric

Student name: _____   **Date:** _____

1 = unsatisfactory, 3 = satisfactory, 5 = exceptional

Patient Care Dimension	Comments: Strengths and Areas for Improvement
INTRODUCTION: Greeted patient, introduced self, verified patient name, used open invitation to talk, smooth opening overall. 1 3 5	
PRIME QUESTIONS: Asked all three questions during encounter.* 1 3 5	
PURPOSE: Explained (or assured understanding of) the purpose of the medication(s). 1 3 5	
GOALS OF THERAPY: Properly communicates goals of therapy for the medication. Describes what response to expect, when to expect response. 1 3 5	
GENERAL DRUG INFO: Told the patient the name, strength, and frequency of administration for the medication or reinforced existing patient knowledge. 1 3 5	
TIMING OF ADMINISTRATION: Explained how to take medication relative to meals or other pertinent daily activities (statins in the evening, bisphosphonates first thing in a.m., etc). 1 3 5	
STORAGE: Explained the proper means of storing the medication. 1 3 5	

Source: Courtesy of Northeast Ohio Medical University College of Pharmacy, Rootstown, OH.

Patient Care Dimension	Comments: Strengths and Areas for Improvement
SIDE EFFECTS: Described the most common/ clinically significant <u>side effects</u> for each medication. 1 3 5	
DURATION/FOLLOW UP: Told the patient <u>how long</u> to take the medication, what to do if <u>a dose is missed</u>, and <u>who to contact</u> if symptoms continue, worsen, and/or there are side effects. 1 3 5	
EXIT: Communicated end of counseling session, gave patient a chance to ask questions and responded appropriately, ended effectively. 1 3 5	

*Prime questions: "What did your doctor tell you about this medication?"; "How did the doctor tell you to take it?"; "What response do you expect to receive from this medication?"

Total score   _____
                                              (maximum score = 50)

Additional comments:

Chapter 7

Dealing with Difficult Situations

Stacey R. Schneider

CASE STUDY

MF is a new preceptor. As a student, she was at the top of the class and on every rotation she strived to perform to the best of her ability. She was always eager for new opportunities and went the extra mile to produce exceptional work. MF is having difficulty relating to learners who do not perform to that same caliber.

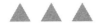

INTRODUCTION

No matter the amount of planning or the caliber of the learners, difficult situations are bound to arise in the course of precepting students and residents. This chapter identifies a number of frequently encountered situations and will provide you with some tips and tools to navigate some of the most common uncomfortable conversations that occur during a rotation.

PROFESSIONALISM

The teaching of professionalism and its maintenance is a hot topic in the profession of pharmacy and across numerous other fields, as well. The difficulty encountered in this area may stem from students being unprepared to exhibit professional behavior or, perhaps, it may ari_____ _____ ___ unclear and inconsistent expectations of professional behavior. _____ when someone is acting in an unprof_____ articulate what professionalism mean_____ n is not, rather than what it is. Ther_____ or.[1-4] Most will include putting the ne_____ ional, providing expert advice in your_____ by your profes- sion while acting with_____ nal is considered by society to be an au_____ f the profession, professional educatio_____ ng. To maintain this expertise, the ind_____ des developing a system to balance the_____ , health, and any other activities of da_____

The most power_____ tudents and resi- dents is through a m_____ round your prac- tice environment. Su_____ and competence. Is your space clean, organized, ___ _____ us to one another and the patients? Is their appearance and demeanor professional? The physical layout and other characteristics of your practice site go a long way in promoting the level of professionalism in your practice. Every student who experiences your rotation will absorb the image you are projecting. Before you can effectively correct professionalism issues, you should ensure you are modeling the proper behaviors.

Is emotional intelligence integral to professionalism? The behaviors cited as manifestations of professionalism are often taught to enhance emotional intelligence. Remember our discussion from Chapter 5 on emotional intelligence, where it was defined as a type of cognitive skill involving the ability to perceive, use, understand, and manage emotion? In a professional environment, where everyday work is emotionally charged, emotional intelligence enhances one's ability to deliver safe and compassionate healthcare. Therefore, it seems that emotional intelligence is a necessary and, perhaps, critical component to teach the concepts of what it means to be a professional.

When you encounter a learner who is struggling with professionalism issues, a good suggestion is to require the student to use reflection to examine his or her emotional response to the situation.[5] Learners will typically arrive prepared with a working knowledge of what constitutes professional behavior. When they act unprofessionally, it is usually the result of a blind spot or extenuating circumstance that brought about the unpleasant behavior. Through the process of self-awareness (a critical component of emotional intelligence), the student can learn to manage emotions internally (self-management) to improve his or her reaction in future situations. After reflecting, the root of the problem may become clearer to the student (and the preceptor), such as a feeling of pressure to answer questions on the spot or a lack of confidence. Once the source of the unprofessional behavior is identified, the preceptor and the learner can work to overcome the underlying issue.

> ## Case Question
>
> *MF has a student who has been rounding with her each morning. She has observed some disturbing behavior from the student, and she is unsure how to approach the situation. She notes the responses the student gives are often short-tempered and frustrated when a team member asks him a question during clinical rounds. How should MF handle this professionalism issue?*

e-Technology, Tools, and Tips

The latest in technology brings much pleasure and productivity to students and professionals alike, but it can come with consequences, as well. We teach our students how to be professional in interviews, at social functions, and in practice settings; however, what happens in cyberspace may not meet the same standard. e-Professionalism involves the same set of behaviors that reflect traditional professionalism but is manifested in digital media. It goes beyond online communication, encompassing the entire online persona of an individual based on the meaning of their online postings, interactions, blogs, images, videos, tweets, and more. When encountering e-professionalism issues, remind students that professional behavior does not stop at the front door of the practice site.

Tips to ensure appropriate communication and online behavior include the following[2]:

- Don't assume that keeping your profile settings private will prevent employers from seeing them
- Check friends' profiles on a regular basis to monitor what pictures and comments are being posted about you
- Don't put anything about your preceptor in a blog or other written posts
- Do a regular online search of your name
- Treat your e-mails like professional correspondence, using correct grammar and only saying those things you would say to someone face to face
- Write your email first and then fill in the recipients' name to avoid sending emails to the wrong destination or before you've completed a review of its contents

To increase the likelihood of professional behavior, provide clear language that specifically describes the required behaviors during the rotation orientation. A creative way to do this may be to ask students to define their professional expectations during the rotation. This will allow for meaningful dialogue and also create buy-in from students, because they are actively involved in the process.

Some examples of professional objectives include the following[2]:

♦ To engage in self-assessment processes
♦ To take accountability for one's own work
♦ To engage in focused, organized, and articulate communication
♦ To negotiate with others assertively and respectfully
♦ To use time management strategies
♦ To display appropriate clothing, language, and mannerisms
♦ To accept and apply constructive criticism

There are tools available to evaluate professional behavior, such as the Behavioral Professionalism Assessment Form.[6] Additionally, role-modeling professionalism goes beyond patient care. Students also learn from the preceptor who is actively engaging in professional organizations, community activities, continuing education, and establishing a healthy work-life balance.

It is difficult to come up with standard tips to handle professional issues. Each situation and learner is different and professionalism issues can happen for a multitude of reasons. The preceptor must be tuned-in to the circumstances, the environment, and the learner.

Here are some general tips to handle a student with professionalism issues:

♦ Sit down and talk to the learner. He or she may have no idea that his or her behavior is a problem. A simple discussion, in which the learner is told there is an issue, may immediately eliminate the problem.
♦ It is essential to explicitly discuss the problematic behavior, explain why it is unacceptable, and reinforce that it will not be tolerated in the future.
♦ In some cases, you may consider beginning progressive discipline depending on the significance of the issue. This may include a verbal warning, written reprimand, and progressing to failure of the rotation.

Do not fall into the trap of making excuses for behavior by thinking it is just a part of the learner's personality. You have every right to demand a professional environment at your site, and it is your responsibility to ensure all learners behave in a manner that is considered respectful and professional.

TIME MANAGEMENT AND PRIORITIZATION ISSUES

Poor time management can lead to chronic procrastination, feelings of incompetence, a sense of isolation, and poor performance. The word *management* implies a conscious level of decision-making. There are a set number of hours in each day and a set number of minutes in each hour; this is completely out of our control. In reality, we cannot manage time. Considering this, time management really means *self-management*. In other words, we monitor ourselves to make the most of time. This involves setting priorities, making a schedule, and monitoring progress. The struggle of time management is not simply a case of cutting back or acquiring new skills, because the exhaustion and fatigue we feel impacts so many areas of life, both personal and professional. This will start to become apparent to you as a preceptor when the student fails to perform to the best of his or her abilities.

Procrastination is the most common student time management problem. Many students, particularly those who found undergraduate course work easy, arrive at rotation sites with efficient procrastination skills. Undoing years of habitual procrastination is not easy, but it can be done. The first step is to understand the reason behind procrastination.

The following suggestions may help you determine why your learner procrastinates and give advice on how to remedy it:

♦ Consider suggesting a journal to help learners become aware of any habits or rituals they are doing that may add to procrastination.

♦ Ask them to list what things motivate and demotivate them.

♦ Encourage them to increase reliance on motivators that are within their control and to remove those factors that decrease motivation.

♦ Guide your learners through a reality check on the goals and expectations they have placed on themselves. If the bar is too high, delays are likely to occur. Not meeting goals often leads to disappointment, guilt, and self-blame, which may further propel the cycle of procrastination.

Tasks that are large and open-ended can be overwhelming to the learner and leave him or her wondering where to start, which just adds to the procrastination. Consider providing periodic checkpoints for bigger projects to help break tasks down into smaller, more manageable pieces so it becomes less stressful for the learner. Set SMART (specific, measurable, attainable, realistic, and timely) goals. You can work with your learners to help figure out the type of tasks they are putting off and if there is a particular time of day they are likely to procrastinate. This will allow the procrastinators to gain insight into how to adjust their use of time and to discover the best environment and hours for personal productivity. Once this is determined, help the learners plan a schedule with the highest priority task occurring during their peak productivity time.

We are each refreshed and restored in different ways, so it is essential to discover which activities drain and which renew our energy levels. Balancing work and personal lives—a real issue for students—can help ensure they are taking time to de-stress. Encourage your learner to think about what they enjoy doing. Stress that they allow themselves the right (without guilt) to do things they enjoy, even if it does not feel as important as professional obligations. Put it on a schedule, if necessary. One of the most valuable things I learned is that doing nothing on my day off is sometimes the most important use of my time! As always, merely acting as a role model as an efficient time manager serves as a great start for the learners around you.

Quick Tip

Begin the first day of the week by asking your learners, "What did you do to relax this weekend?" This helps to reinforce the importance of down-time.

UNPREPARED LEARNERS

It is difficult to teach if students are unprepared to learn. It is crucial to investigate what could be happening in this scenario. Are there barriers to learning? Perhaps the student did not study in a way that led him or her to retain information. Many students memorize facts but are not able to use critical thinking. At this point in their training, one hopes it is not due to a lack of motivation or effort. Asking the right questions will help you figure out the cause of the unpreparedness.

If you see that the student is unprepared, it is a good idea to assess his or her clinical baseline knowledge so you know where the gaps are and how to fill them. You may have to change your objectives for the rotation if you learn there are essential knowledge gaps. To increase knowledge about clinical decisions, discuss cases and use them as a way to discuss disease topics, as a whole. In other words, the student does not only investigate all the elements of the particular case, but the preceptor changes the case in a way that challenges the student to draw on knowledge of the other facets of the disease state. Asking the right questions will encourage the student to develop critical thinking skills. Change the case dynamics of the case using "what if" questions. *What if* the age of the patient changed? *What if* our first recommendation did not work? Using these teaching points to help the student work through different scenarios allows for reviews of the disease state presented.

Whereas knowledge base may be the issue in some cases, unprepared learners can also be struggling with time management. This occurs more often with a more advanced learner, such as a resident who has had more time to develop his or her clinical skills. If this is the case, consider how to help the learner improve time management skills as described in the section above.

If time management is not the issue, perhaps the student is afraid to give answers in a large group. An introverted student needs more time to process knowledge before responding. In this case, you should give the student an opportunity to look up information ahead of time to allow him or her to digest the information and develop a response. Not answering in front of others may also be a self-confidence issue. In this case, students usually know the answers but do not trust themselves enough to speak up. You will need to spend time with the student one-on-one to go through various critical thinking exercises to give positive feedback when the student is on the right track. In this way, the student will begin to see he or she actually knows the right answers. With each bit of positive feedback, the learner's confidence will increase. As learners get more practice in voicing their recommendations, they will be more likely to speak up, trusting that they have the correct answers.

Quick Tip

It is essential to create a safe learning environment when learners are introverted or lack self-confidence. A student who feels safe making mistakes with you is likely to find their own voice and come out of their shell.

ENTITLED LEARNERS

There are many reasons entitlement happens in society. Some learners are accustomed to being rewarded for participating, not producing. For others, failure may have been eschewed to avoid damaging self-esteem. The concept of the student as a consumer may also play a role, leading some to believe that the customer is always right, allowing some students to blame others for their own failures. Academic entitlement may spill over from the classroom, affecting what preceptors see at the practice site.

Some red flag behaviors you may encounter include the following:

♦ Students who provide excuses when poor work is submitted
♦ Students who expect high grades regardless of their performance
♦ Students who expect all learning to be delivered from the preceptor without significant effort on their part as learners[7]

Entitlement will not go away easily. Instead, preceptors should put a process in place to lead them from entitlement to empowerment. You may have authority, but you must earn your influence by building your students' trust

The following are some tips to eliminate entitlement:

♦ *Be a good role model.* If you embody the attitude and work ethic you demand of your students, you will start disarming an entitled student.
♦ *Communicate clearly the deadlines and guidelines for work assignments and do not compromise.* If you do give in to demands, you can actually create a deepened sense of entitlement as your rules are manipulated.
♦ *Do not discuss rules.* Focus, instead, on consequences for not meeting expectations. Students need to learn to live with behavioral consequences.
♦ *Relay to your students that failure is not an end-all.* Establish an environment where it is safe to fail. If you remove the fear of failure, they just may allow themselves to struggle through the learning process and become better practitioners as a result. Failure can actually be viewed as very positive and, perhaps, one of the many ways to learn and grow personally and professionally.

In these situations, it becomes even more important to document every incident and report them to the experiential director at the time of occurrence. As you work through issues of entitlement, communicating the issues as they occur protects you from backlash or claims of discrimination. Waiting until the end of the rotation will benefit no one.

Case Question

MF was excited to precept her first resident, but the experience was significantly different than her own residency. Instead of going the extra mile, the resident seemed to sit back and wait for MF to do all of the teaching. The resident did not participate actively in topic discussions or seek feedback for her performance. List two steps MF could take to empower her resident to take ownership in her own development.

DISINTERESTED LEARNERS

You will eventually come in contact with a student who is not interested in your rotation. It is hard to feel your time is not being wasted. There are a few things you can do to avoid this: (1) provide as much information as possible for students prior to selecting the rotation; (2) give enough insight so there is a good idea of what opportunities and learning experiences your site will provide. This will let them know what to expect prior to the rotation and can assure a good match. When a student does not know what to expect, his or her demeanor may express disinterest but may likely be due to apprehension with the unexpected.

Before starting your rotation, ask learners about previous experiences and what they want to learn from you or why they chose your rotation. This will allow for customization of your learning experience to match the needs and goals of the learner. Ask them to help provide objectives to gauge their interest and needs. This allows them the opportunity to be vested in the learning experience. Let students know what their positions are in relation to the medical team. If they are not clear on their role, the uncertainty may lead to what appears as disinterest, as well. Knowledge base issues may also present as an apparent disinterest in the rotation and will require you to spend time identifying knowledge gaps and modifying your objectives to fix these gaps. Lack of adequate feedback can lead to disinterest, as well, leading students to think you are not interested in them. Learners are hungry for your feedback, and continuous feedback helps to encourage a less confident student once they see they are improving.

To help you connect with your learner, spend some time with him or her, such as a coffee break or a lunch hour. This may help you understand the student's motivations and the source of disinterest. Spending this extra time lets the student know you are interested in his or her learning. These sessions may help you uncover distressing things going on in the learner's personal life. You can open the lines of communication with genuine concern for their well-being and his or her performance on your rotation. This may give your student the opportunity to open up to you and ask for help. It is advisable to be aware of the resources your site or school provides to aid your student before having this conversation.

Students who sense a disconnect between what they are learning and their future career are unlikely to engage to the same degree as students who understand the relevant connections between current learning and their future. If you want to increase the level of engagement, you must demonstrate how the skills they learn on your rotation will be applicable to their future practice. This can be done throughout the rotation. How many times have I heard, "Why do I have to do internal medicine if I want to practice in the community?" Once I helped the student to see that we were encountering the same disease states and patients that are seen in the community, learning began to take place. Learners can also sense when you are passionate about what you teach, and the feeling cannot help but be contagious. If you make learning fun and exciting for them, it may be enough to convert a disinterested learner into an interested one.

OVERCONFIDENT LEARNERS

Overconfidence can be a real problem for learners. It can cause a student to experience problems related to improper preparation, or they may find themselves in a situation that they are not equipped to handle. When they are sure they have got it right, they do not try to improve their understanding. This leads to not checking facts that can lead to disastrous consequences for the student, other colleagues, as well as patients.

The overconfident student may display an overinflated sense of worth, lack of empathy, or a desire for attention. While they seem very content, they can rely heavily on the appreciation and approval of others t(

stem from the fact that a student had a great d

ous experiences or has not been challenged to

her accustomed to succeeding and leads to the

You will need to be cautious with overconfi

al, as they will usually react badly to criticism

criticize them in an attempt to bring their ego b

a peg." Start by explaining that they are still l

their overconfidence has affected patient care.

humility and make them aware of the conseq

to give on-the-spot feedback each time they ju

by exploring the topic in a way that helps the

brought to their attention in this manner, you

identify a flaw of which they were previously

the idea if the redirection is done in this manner. You may also try another tactic, such

as the *sandwich technique*. This is commonly used when giving constructive feedback.

It translates to one negative statement in between two positive statements. This helps to

soften the blow while still delivering the crucial feedback that these learners need.

Case Question

MF started a new rotation with a student who was very quick to jump in when counseling patients. The student hit the ground running from day one and was not afraid to voice her clinical opinion. However, on multiple occasions MF found flaws in what the student was suggesting to the patient. When confronted about the errors, the student would assume that MF misunderstood her or brushed off the criticism by saying, "Oh yeah, that's what I meant to say, but I phrased it wrong." How should MF approach the subject so that the student takes the critique to heart and improves her patient care skills?

COMMUNICATION ISSUES

With the increasing diversity in our society, it is likely at one time or another we will all precept a student with English as a second language (ESL). Teaching ESL students can be challenging, frustrating, and require a lot of resources. Before tackling the educational piece, you must consider the ESL learner's social, emotional, and developmental needs. First and foremost, all preceptors should take a moment to reflect on their own knowledge in regard to cultural differences. Take the time to learn about different cultures and traditions and celebrate the need for diversity in our profession.

Secondly, empathize with the ESL student by trying to imagine how overwhelming it must feel to leave your home country while trying to learn and socialize in a foreign language. Use patience and understand that it will take time for ESL students to adjust. Taking time to become culturally competent and empathize with your ESL student will place you far ahead in the precepting process.

When a student first arrives on your rotation, get to know as much possible about him or her. ESL students can arrive with a wide range of academic skills, interests, languages, English language proficiency, and cultures. The more you can learn about the student's background, the better prepared you will be to precept that student. Your expectations should not change for students who are still developing English language skills. Creative teachers think of ways to help students understand key material and show competency in ways that match their language proficiency levels.

Encourage the ESL student to socialize with other students or residents, such as during lunchtime, to help provide opportunities to practice the language in an informal setting. Also, encourage them to join groups where they will be challenged by those of different cultures instead of remaining in a safe zone. ESL students must recognize the importance of exposing themselves to English in natural settings. Students who tend to function primarily in their native language in their personal lives are at a disadvantage when compared to others who use the English language outside of educational settings, such as watching television, listening to music, reading newspapers, or conversing with people they meet in public. During your rotation, provide as many opportunities as possible for talking and listening to others, either with one-on-one discussion or in small group discussions. In small groups, students are more likely to verbalize, allowing the ESL learners to practice both their English language skills and their clinical skills.

When giving tasks to students, specifically model what you expect them to do. In other words, show them how to accomplish the task and give an example of exactly how the final product should look, such as showing them an example of how to deliver a journal club or case presentation rather than just presenting them with a grading rubric. Once again, modeling behavior becomes invaluable. When engaged in discussions, provide sufficient response time for ESL students. They are hearing what you say in English and they may need to think of the words in their native language to truly process what has been said. Then they will decide on a response in their native language, adapt that response to their English vocabulary, think about the response to make sure that it makes sense, and, finally, respond. It often takes years of exposure to the English language before a student can bypass the translation steps and truly think in English.

Fear of failure and embarrassment are quite common and can be debilitating. To these students, learning becomes frightening, and isolation seems safest. If you get the sense that a student is persistently isolating or withdrawing for fear of using English, you must get involved immediately. In the case of a student for whom fear has become an obstacle to learning, some personalized attention from the preceptor can help. This allows the student to develop trust in the preceptor, which is a form of social support that may be missing if the ESL student does not have family in the area.

I learned this firsthand when an ESL student told me that she was fearful of speaking up in class because her classmates would make fun of her accent. She was having an extremely difficult time communicating with patients, as well. I saw the translation process of converting English language to her native language, formulating a thought, then translating it back again to English to respond to the patient. That alone must have been exhausting for the student! I called her into my office, desperate to help her with communication skills. She told me at home she only spoke in her native language to her family and read printed materials in her native language. We came up with a plan to meet weekly to have a discussion about an article she read in a magazine. I encouraged her not to pick scientific reading but something that was enjoyable for her and taught her more about our culture. We did this on a continuous basis for a few months. I questioned her when I did not understand what she was trying to relay and, in the process, helped to form her communication skills. The student went on to be very successful in the curriculum. In essence, I provided her a safe place and the social support of a professor who truly believed she had the skills to be successful.

There is no quick fix, course, or textbook that can be used for teaching ESL, and no two students will be alike. Language learning depends on age, background, interests, previous schooling and current needs. Expecting errors and having patience is key in the learning process. Remember that it is imperative to provide a safe and supportive environment to enhance second language learning.

THE FAST LEARNER

Keeping quick learners engaged can often be exhausting and feels, at times, like a struggle. Assignments are turned in early, extra learning experiences may be sought, and it can be difficult to come up with new challenges. On the upside, these students are so driven, passionate, and hungry for knowledge that it can be exhilarating for the preceptor.

The key to precepting fast learners is to motivate them and make them feel valued. From the beginning of the rotation, you will realize that your fast learners may need little guidance and encourage them to make clinical decisions on their own (with your oversight). These students desire to feel valued as a relevant part of the team and want their knowledge base to be used. What happens if you do not agree? The solution is to focus on the evidence and not the opinion. As you focus on the science, begin to formulate clinical questions, look up data together, and talk through the data to find an agreeable solution. Valuing learners' input lets them know they are an integral and important part of the decision-making process.

Teach your gifted learners how to apply information, which is the key to clinical practice. Fast learners may have the extensive knowledge base but may need the preceptor to help guide them toward critical thinking and application of materials. Also, challenge them to use their knowledge to teach others. Teaching a subject usually requires mastering the material, further solidifying the learner's knowledge base. Encourage learners to give presentations to other students, colleagues, and staff. This will help polish their communication skills and, in turn, likely increase the knowledge of you and your staff.

Having an excellent student is a win for all parties. If you are not feeling confident when you have a gifted learner, sit back and reflect on your own practice and give yourself time to discover why this is occurring. Perhaps you are deficient in your knowledge base? Perhaps you are very proficient in your own practice but less familiar areas could use some brushing up. Be humble enough to let your fast learner educate you as well as your staff. After all, having him or her on rotation should be a beneficial situation for everyone.

PERSONALITY ISSUES AND BIASES

No matter how you characterize your personality, you should appreciate not everyone is like you. People are inherently and genetically different. When we understand the people around us, we will become successful at forming healthy relationships. Imagine working with people exactly like you. Wouldn't that get rather boring? Different personalities can be constructive for a workplace because they allow for many different opinions and ideas. There are those who are enthusiastic, funny, and loud. They are extroverts who love talking, often speaking before (or while) they think. There are those who are assertive, decisive, and productive. They are the ones always taking control and getting things done. These people are meticulous and work to create structure, order, and compliance. Then there are those who are easy-going, diplomatic, and patient. They hate conflict and do everything in their power to avoid confrontation. They do not have highs or lows, and are often hard to read. Isn't it to the benefit of an organization to employ people with all of these different strengths? You must surround yourself with colleagues of different strengths and experiences to build a solid team, as well as to learn and grow.

As a preceptor, you need to learn to be tolerant and accepting of other personalities. You can do this once you realize that most people are merely products of their personality types and experiences. Through mutual understanding, you can get along with just about anyone. Consider that vast differences may be generational or cultural. Get to know your students early in the rotation so you may get to know them as people rather than students, helping to establish a mutual respect between you and students. If you know what makes them tick, you will better understand how they act in certain situations.

One source of personality clash may result from your student's learning style not matching your teaching style. Each of us has our own natural style of thinking, processing information, problem solving, and communicating. By learning to give the other person the information he or she needs in the manner he or she can process it most efficiently, you can create a productive learning environment. You need to be open-minded and flexible enough to change your teaching style to meet your student's needs.

To overcome personality differences, you must respect your student or resident. Only by giving respect will you get it back. Learn to appreciate individual strengths. Learning more about different personality types will help you understand and appreciate others. It is also useful to step into their shoes and imagine what it is like for them. How do they view the world? And how do they view you? Keep reminding yourself that they are not being difficult, they are just being themselves. Be aware of your own weaknesses. It helps the situation if we realize that our personality type has its own weaknesses and pitfalls that might rankle others! There is no perfect personality type, just personality differences.

Discover how to motivate your learners and what is important to them while on your rotation. Blend this into your objectives and strike a balance between students' needs and your rotation's objectives. Do *not* compromise your rotation to please the student. One of the most valuable words of advice a seasoned faculty member gave me was "You are not here to be their friend. However, you may hope that from their interactions with you they leave as better pharmacists."

THE EMOTIONAL LEARNER

Not so long ago, emotions were considered to be obstacles to productivity in the workplace. We were told to leave them at the door once we got to work. Although this attitude still exists, most of us recognize that our emotions are part of who we are, and we may have no choice but to bring them to work. But the question now becomes, how do we deal with them once we are at work? At times, everyone has to deal with negative emotions at work, and learning how to cope with these feelings is a valuable skill to teach your students.

At the beginning of the rotation as you set up your professional expectations, discuss how the student is expected to handle emotional situations. Depending on your site, discuss some emotional experiences they may encounter. Perhaps it is a disgruntled customer, an angry colleague, or situations involving death and dying. The more prepared the students are, the better they will be able to handle their emotions. It may be helpful if you describe how you learned to deal with your emotions when encountering these situations for the first time. Establish yourself as a safe person to talk to. You can prevent public displays of emotions if the learners know they can come to you when they have overwhelming emotions.

An emotionally intelligent person will investigate what is causing negative emotions and which types of feelings are surfacing most often. It may be anger, fear, worry, frustration, or a number of other emotions. When those emotions begin to appear, stop and evaluate the situation to understand why those emotions are occurring. It may help if you write down specifics about the situation. Depending on the emotion, immediately start a strategy to interrupt the cycle. This may be deep breathing, thinking of the positives instead of the negatives of the situation, or figuring out how to improve the situation. As a preceptor, you can help the student work through this process and help to find acceptable strategies to diffuse the emotion. For example, if the student becomes overwhelmed with anger, make it acceptable to leave the situation. Sometimes these emotions become so strong that the best way to deal with them is to leave a situation until we get our emotions under control.

Crying can happen for numerous reasons, either personal or professional. Crying is a biological function of our lacrimal glands and autonomic nervous system. We are rarely in charge when we cry. Once the crying reflex gets triggered, most of us are helpless to stop it. Perhaps an intense empathetic situation results in crying. The response to the death of a patient may be related to something that happened in the student's life; for example, the death of a family member. There is an appropriate time and place to express this, but it is not appropriate in front of the patient's family. When there are tears, this is a sign that there is an emotion or situation that needs to be dealt with. This can be very therapeutic for your student if handled appropriately and in a private place.

Always use the emotional situation as a learning experience. Talk through how the student handled the issue and discuss how you may have handled the situation differently. As you work through what provoked the emotion, do not make assumptions as to why the emotion occurred. In these types of conversations with your students, it is critical to think before you speak. Your students are listening, and your words are more important to them than you probably realize. As a preceptor approaching an emotional issue with a student, it is important to remain calm, state misconduct, and avoid debating or arguing with the student. Teach students to describe the conflict or problem, identify possible responses, select a response, and evaluate the selected response. You might consider introducing opportunities for free writing or journaling to help the student express his or her feelings.

When do you need to call in help? Perhaps you are not getting the full story or the student has not developed complete trust in you to open up. Before you begin precepting, familiarize yourself with the available resources to help your students. It is acceptable to ask a colleague for advice, but do not use information that would identify the student. Moving forward, it will be necessary to assess whether your environment allows the student to be successful. Can you minimize disruptions and emotional situations? If not, it might require further conversations with the director of the program.

DEALING WITH ERRORS

As supervisors of students and residents, preceptors will need to deal with their trainees' errors. The preceptor will need to be skilled in the teaching and learning that should take place surrounding that error. There are numerous types of errors. Some errors are considered clearly wrong (such as administering the wrong drug), whereas others may be less obvious (such as administering a second-line antibiotic). Some preceptors may view minor errors as beneficial opportunities because the lack of urgency allows time for teaching. Some of your students or residents may brush off errors, and others may try to cover up errors if there was no harm done. This is as a sign of immaturity. Students may experience emotional responses accompanying the error. This ranges from feelings of distress, remorse, shame, incompetence, and self-doubt. Helping the learner deal with these feelings is a prerequisite for a teaching moment to occur. Once an error has been recognized, the learner will likely gain skills or the knowledge that would prevent him or her from making that same error again. Sometimes the new skill or knowledge may be obvious, and at other times it will require instruction from the preceptor.

A necessary first step is to bring the error to the student's attention. Recognizing errors and assuming responsibility is the first step to learning from the error. Ideally, you hope your student takes this step without your direction; but, in some cases, the preceptor will need to encourage the learner to take responsibility. The next step is to examine the path to the error. This is best accomplished in a one-on-one discussion. Verify that the student understands why certain procedures are necessary or integral in preventing future errors, such as reviewing all of the checkpoints required to verify prescriptions. If the error was due to a lack of knowledge, then having the student review appropriate guidelines, textbooks, or journal articles would be appropriate.

Some preceptors may find that teaching from their own errors is helpful. This may actually be a way to prevent errors by conveying the importance of practices that seem to be mundane to learners who have not had to experience the consequences of an error. This is also a good way to model your actions as a result of the error. This will help the student see how to work through what caused the error and how to take responsibility in all situations.

Attention to emotional support for students may be necessary in some cases. Reassurance will help the student realize that errors happen to all healthcare providers, and the most important lesson is how to avoid them in the future. You can also investigate your own actions: if you did not provide enough guidance or supervision, take responsibility for that and let the student know that you are partially responsible for the error. Avoid anger or harsh reprimands, as these only create a roadblock to learning from the error and may impede the student.

Reflecting on an error requires us to look through an ethical lens. Allowing an incompetent healthcare practitioner to progress in an educational program is a breech of ethical responsibility because it puts future patients at risk and compromises the integrity of the profession. It can also damage the credibility of an educational program. As a preceptor, it is your responsibility to ensure the clinical competence of your student or resident and evaluate his or her performance. When faced with evaluating a student who is not meeting practice standards, there is a great deal of extra work involved. This ranges from discussing the issue with the student, other faculty, and the director of the program to developing a plan that allows an opportunity for the student to show improvement. Of course, clear documentation must be an ongoing process. Compassion for the student is important, but equally important is compassion for the patients. The reality is that the preceptor has two options: allowing progression or assigning a failing grade. If the practices of the student threaten patient safety and compromise the integrity of the profession, the preceptor must do the right thing and report the unsafe student and assign a failing grade. When in doubt, it may help to ask "Would I want this student taking care of one of my family members?" or "Would I want to work with this student?" If these questions bring forth a negative response, it is the preceptor's ethical responsibility to fail the student.

As a preceptor, you are a teacher and, therefore, should expect errors as part of the learning process. There is always a chance for medical errors to occur simply because of the human element in healthcare. It is your responsibility to address these errors. Avoid common barriers such as lack of time or lack of a private space. If an error occurs in a public place, set time aside to have a private conversation with the student as soon as possible. It takes a skilled preceptor to learn how to deal not only with the behavioral implications of a medical error but also the emotional response to the error. In all cases, be aware of your site's procedures for reporting errors and comply with the regulations set forth by your institution.

Case Question

While completing their staffing requirement, one of MF's residents skipped a few steps in the order verification process when the pharmacy was particularly busy. As a result, an error was made, and the wrong medication was dispensed to a patient. What is the best way the MF should go about handling this situation?

BALANCING GIFTED AND STRUGGLING LEARNERS

We have talked about so many different types of students and situations you will encounter. Think how good it would be to get two students who were basically similar. Life as a preceptor would be much easier if each student arrived with the same knowledge and skill base, same learning style, same strengths and weaknesses. However, we do not live in a perfect world. You will likely never have a perfect match when trying to teach multiple learners. All students are different in terms of their achievement, ability, learning and cognitive styles, as well as attitudes, pace of learning, personality, and motivation. Adapting instruction to each student's skills and needs while advancing learning for all students is no small feat.

Students will likely have different learning styles. You need to consider how learners perceive, interact with, and respond to the environment around them. Learning styles can be influenced by personality and culture. Auditory learners need to hear information in order to learn. If you have an auditory learner, you need to talk through concepts. Visual learners need to see the information to learn. For these types of learners, using tables, figures, and diagrams as a teaching method can be particularly useful. There are learners who need to see the big picture, whereas others need to break down the big picture into smaller concepts before making connections. Some of your learners will learn more effectively in groups, whereas others are highly successful through individual learning. Help learners identify their styles so they will be able to focus and use their method of learning.

What if the learning style is not a match with the teaching style? Even if the teaching and learning style is a perfect match, there are still pros and cons to consider. If everything matches, the students will learn easily. However, easy learning could facilitate entitlement, because it gives the students material in the format they prefer. This may prevent students from adapting to other types of learning. In the real world, students may not get information in the manner they desire and become frustrated. Hence, there is great benefit to having a mismatch and forcing students to shift gears and adapt. Because you cannot be expected to match every student's preferred learning style, and mismatches can foster growth and adaptation, the key will be to simply avoid teaching in only one style. It takes a skilled preceptor to use different teaching styles. Give yourself time to practice and adjust your teaching style when you have different types of learners.

At times, you may be assigned students at completely different levels. How do you separate them and give them different responsibilities without highlighting the fast versus struggling learner? Would this create a mental setback in the one who was struggling? Requiring both of them to do the same activities will benefit neither learner nor push them to their maximum potential. If the struggling learner is pushed into activities in which he or she lacks the basic skills and knowledge to perform, he or she will be anxious and uncomfortable and not benefit from the rotation. Engaging fast learners in activities that bore them would likely breed disinterest, disappointment, and frustration.

In this case, the best approach is to reexamine and modify the objectives for the struggling learner and assign different opportunities for both students. Coming back together for group discussions is paramount. They will challenge each other in different ways. The struggling student can look to the fast student for tips on how to be successful, and the fast student can be challenged to teach a struggling student. To flip the role of the teacher to the fast student is a benefit in itself, pushing learners in ways they have yet to experience through teaching. However, you must be very cautious with how much you empower the fast-learning student to act as the teacher. A sensitive line needs to be drawn so as to not demean a struggling learner, requiring a highly emotionally intelligent fast learner.

So what does this mean when you change your expectations for the different types of students? Does the challenged learner fail because he or she is not able to meet the same expectations as the fast learner? Not necessarily. The preceptor must feel comfortable with the fact that students will have very different personalities, opportunities, needs, and objectives for future careers. As long as the basic requirements for your rotation are met, the struggling learner can earn a passing grade. You must adjust your mindset to allow both students to excel. Take the opportunity to assess each student's strengths and guide them through a career development process. Focus on the different strengths of each student and relay that differing strengths does not mean weaker versus stronger or intelligent versus less intelligent. Rather, it means we all have different strengths that are waiting to be uncovered and used to the best of our ability to help determine our most beneficial path in life.

Case Question

During her latest advanced pharmacy practice experience rotation, MF is faced with two drastically different learners with different levels of experience, knowledge, skills, learning styles, personalities, self-confidence, and emotional maturity. In the past, both learners have been equally matched, or at least close enough so that they were able to work together. After 1 week it became clear that this was not going to work in this case. How can MF serve the needs of both students?

THE GIST

1. Professionalism is reinforced by setting expectations, performing assessments, and remediating inappropriate behaviors.
2. The essential key to dealing with any type of situation is clear, open, and honest communication with the learner.
3. Each student and situation is unique, and it takes a nonbiased, emotionally intelligent, compassionate preceptor to turn the worst situation into a positive learning experience for a learner.

SUGGESTED READING

Berger BA. *Communication Skills for Pharmacists*. Washington, DC: American Pharmacists Association; 2011.

Davis LE, Miller ML, Raub JN et al. Constructive ways to prevent, identify, and remediate deficiencies of "challenging trainees" in experiential education. *Am J Health-Syst Pharm.* 2016; 73:996-1109.

Purkerson Hammer D, Mason HL, Chalmers RK et al. Development and testing of an instrument to assess behavioral professionalism of pharmacy students. *Am J Pharm Educ.* 2000; 62:141-51.

REFERENCES

1. Hammer D. Improving student professionalism during experiential learning. *Am J Pharm Educ.* 2006; 70(3):59.

2. American Pharmacists Association–Academy of Student Pharmacists–American Association of Colleges of Pharmacy Committee on Student Professionalism. Pharmacy professionalism toolkit for students and faculty (2009). http://www.aacp.org/resources/studentaffairspersonnel/studentaffairspolicies/Documents/Version_2%200_Pharmacy_Professionalism_Toolkit_for_Students_and_Faculty.pdf. Accessed July 17, 2016.

3. Chalmers RK. Contemporary issues: professionalism in pharmacy. *Tomorrows Pharm.* 1997; March:10-2.

4. American College of Clinical Pharmacy. Tenets of professionalism for pharmacy students. *Pharmacotherapy.* 2009; 29:757-9.

5. Nuffer W, Vaughn J, Kerr K et al. A three-year reflective writing program as part of introductory pharmacy practice experiences. *Am J Pharm Educ.* 2013; 77(5):100.

6. Purkerson Hammer D, Mason HL, Chalmers RK et al. Development and testing of an instrument to assess behavioral professionalism of pharmacy students. *Am J Pharm Educ.* 2000; 62:141-51.

7. Brukner H. Giving effective feedback to medical students: a workshop for faculty and house staff. *Med Teach.* 1999; 21:161-5.

Chapter 8

Wrapping Up the Rotation

S. Scott Wisneski

CASE STUDY

SW is Director of Pharmacy Operations at a community teaching hospital currently precepting SS, who is completing a 4-week management elective advanced pharmacy practice experience (APPE). SS has indicated to SW that she is interested in pursuing a career in hospital pharmacy management. SW completes the final evaluation for SS, indicating that she performed very well, meeting all the rotation objectives. SW provides some general comments reflecting SS's positive performance but also states, "SS's interpersonal skills need substantial development if she plans to pursue a career in management." While SW is going over the evaluation, SS is surprised about the comment and feels she did quite well on the rotation. She is concerned that this comment may impact her chances of pursing a residency and career in pharmacy management. SW states that some of the staff pharmacists and technicians indicated that she seemed cold and unwilling to interact with them. He could provide no further details related to these comments from the staff, and he was already late for a meeting. SS leaves the rotation visibly upset.

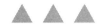

INTRODUCTION

As the end of a rotation approaches, you will undoubtedly need to prepare and deliver a final evaluation of the experience to your student or resident. Because this is almost always associated with the assignment of a grade, these summative assessments can be crucial to your students' future plans. A good grade can help a pharmacy student obtain a residency position or a resident obtain his or her desired postgraduate year (PGY) 2 residency. On the other hand, a nonpassing grade could delay a student's graduation or delay the next step of a resident's career. You may feel pressured to provide a positive evaluation, but you also have a duty to ensure one has demonstrated the skills necessary to be a competent pharmacy professional. Passing a student who does not possess the knowledge and skill to become an independent practitioner could lead to patient harm. Thus, issuing a failing grade is in the best interest not just of the student but patients and the profession, as well. This warrants spending adequate time preparing and presenting a final evaluation to your student or resident.

PREPARING A FINAL EVALUATION

Preparation for the final evaluation really begins long before the student starts the rotation. You need to review and understand how they will be assessed. Schools or colleges of pharmacy and residency programs will have specific rotation criteria, evaluation forms, and grading procedures you should review. It is important to know what specific evaluation parameters (such as "exceeding expectations," "progressing satisfactorily," "achieved objectives," and "needs improvement") mean before completing any student assessment. Often, the source of the evaluation will place these definitions on the form itself. Residency programs will typically have a policy document related to resident assessment that could also house this information. You also need to be familiar with what constitutes a passing or failing grade. Appendix 8A is an example of a college of pharmacy's APPE final evaluation.

During the rotation orientation, it is essential that you review the final evaluation process with the students or residents. This discussion should include review of the rotation objectives, how they will be assessed, and expectations for positive performance. Ideally, you would have identified and planned specific activities that one will complete to best assess each objective of the rotation (see Chapter 1). This can include formal presentations, disease state topic discussions, patient work-ups, journal clubs, and other activities that will be assessed to measure performance. Any separate assessment tools or rubrics that you may use to assess the learner's performance of an activity should also be reviewed. See Chapter 6 for more information and examples of these tools. You will want to provide your expectations for given levels of performance, such as honors, meeting expectations, or unsatisfactory performance. If other pharmacists, pharmacy technicians, or healthcare providers will be providing input into the evaluations, this should be discussed, as well. Describe how their comments will be included in the final evaluation. In some cases, it may be direct quotes from the individual or summarized into your own comments. Finally, a date and time for the final evaluation should be determined and added to the student's or resident's rotation calendar. This early discussion helps to ensure the students understand how their final evaluation will be completed, ultimately making the evaluation process run smoother and prevent any confusion for them.

Quick Tip

Have your student prepare a weekly reflection as a method to encourage self-assessment of his or her rotation performance. Collect and review the documents just before you complete your evaluation so you can ensure the student has appropriate self-evaluation skills.

When the end of the rotation arrives, you might find it difficult to remember all of the ways your students did or did not meet expectations. Relying solely on your memory can lead to a mismatch between the students' actual performance and the final assessments you complete. Throughout the rotation, you will be continually evaluating the students' performance. As described in Chapter 6, it is essential for you to provide ongoing formative feedback and a summative evaluation midway during the rotation. This provides the students an ongoing assessment of their performance by identifying areas of strength as well as skills needing further development. Documentation of feedback can ease the final evaluation process. Use of assessment tools targeting key activities, such as case presentations, journal clubs, and drug information questions, can be effective documentation. While gathering up these data points and rubrics, consider collecting evaluations from other preceptors who had opportunities to spend time with your students. Physicians on rounds, technicians in the department, and administrators in meetings can all help provide additional information to make your final evaluation more complete. Another suggestion is to document ongoing performance on a copy of the actual final evaluation form, avoiding the pitfall of having to remember how a student performed on a past activity. This is especially helpful if the preceptor has multiple students present during a given month. Taking the time to routinely assess and document student performance throughout the experience will be helpful when completing the final evaluation.

As the rotation gets closer to completion, ideally during the final week, the preceptor should begin to write the evaluation. It is important to take plenty of time to accurately document and comment on how the students performed during the experience. If the preceptor has been periodically assessing and documenting performance, as described above, writing the final evaluation should be relatively easy. In contrast, waiting until the last hour to collect your thoughts and prepare the assessment will be far less effective. Either way, it is crucial that you objectively complete the assessments, giving full consideration to your students' performance compared with the standards provided in the evaluation forms.

It is important to ensure that the final assessment is based on the overall performance throughout the rotation.[1] Although a student may have had difficulty early on, the final evaluation should reflect his or her progression toward meeting the rotation's objectives. Do not dwell on a single negative incident, especially if the student has made improvements. On the other hand, if the individual failed to make the needed adjustments to demonstrate achievement of certain objectives, the preceptor should clearly indicate this in the final evaluation. Citing specific examples of performance is crucial in these incidents. Preceptors should also be sure to adequately provide positive comments when the student or resident has performed at a level that exceeds expectations. In some cases, the college or school of pharmacy will require to see your written comments justifying an assessment that exceeds expectations. Your comments can further motivate a high achiever and may be used by the student or resident when applying for a residency or job. The final evaluation should also provide feedback on specific areas that need improvement in the future. This helps the individual know what he or she needs to work on during upcoming rotations or prior to starting a career. A common preceptor mistake is to simply list students' completed activities, leaving out any comments on how they performed on a given activity. Those comments are important because the students can use them to further develop their skills. Also, if the evaluation is shared with other preceptors, your comments will be helpful to those individuals as they prepare for the student or resident. Like formative feedback, your comments should reflect the specific behaviors supporting both positive and negative performance and refrain from comments that center on personal traits.

Quick Tip

Provide written comments any time students exceed or do not meet your expectations. The more specific the comment, the more useful it will be.

Case Question

How could SW do a better job providing comments about his student's interpersonal skills?

You may notice a drift toward issuing high marks in many, if not all, of the domains in the final evaluation form, a tendency known as *grade inflation*. This could give the appearance that the preceptor has not taken adequate time to accurately assess each component of the evaluation. Keep in mind that the majority of students will likely have some skills that need further development, and, as such, the final evaluation should appropriately reflect performance in each area assessed during the rotation. While the students may welcome the high marks, it can cause them to incorrectly believe that they need no further development. This leads to confusion when a subsequent preceptor provides a more accurate assessment and a lower grade. The students or residents will be unsure why one preceptor issued high marks while another issued lower scores.

The following tips will help you avoid grade inflation:

- Objectively evaluate each component of the assessment, considering how the student performed.
- Avoid the tendency to look at the final grade to see if the student passed or failed. If you find yourself changing the marks to force a certain final score, you may likely be committing grade inflation.
- Use comments to back up the chosen score. If you are truly being objective, the comments should be easy to write. On the other hand, if you are struggling with providing a comment to justify a score, then reconsider the marks you have provided.

Remember, you are not "giving" a grade. Instead, your job is to indicate the grade the student earned. Using these suggestions can help prevent the tendency to provide inflated scores.

Similar to grade inflation, some preceptors fall victim to the practice of always issuing scores below the maximum a student can earn, a bias that can be described as *undergrading*. This occurs when a preceptor believes no one is capable of a high mark. Avoid this type of predisposition when completing final evaluations. A student or resident who has performed specific aspects of a rotation in an excellent manner deserves the opportunity to receive high marks. As you complete an evaluation, you should carefully assess each area of the student's performance and issue a grade that is in line with the performance you have witnessed. Early consideration of your expectations in each of the areas to be assessed can be helpful in accurately preparing a final evaluation.

The following tips will help you avoid undergrading:

♦ Determine the performance that would actually exceed your expectations for each component of the evaluation. Reflect on past students who performed above your expectations and ask yourself, "What was it that he or she did to perform in such a manner?" This can be used as a guide when assessing future students.

♦ Avoid being too narrow in your definition of exceeded expectations and be open to reconsider how you measure student performance.

♦ Compare your assessment with other preceptors grading similar types of rotations. Schools or colleges of pharmacy can often assist you in creating this type of comparison. If you find your grading is generally lower than your peers, you might want to identify where you may be biased or have set an expectation at an unachievable level.

♦ Consider the stage of the student. The level of performance of an introductory pharmacy practice experiences student is going to be different from one completing an APPE. The same would be true for a PGY1 versus a PGY2 resident. Expectations of performance must align with the type of student or resident being assessed.

Quick Tip

It may be helpful to periodically review the grades you have given for the last six students completing your learning experience. Look for any signs of grade inflation or undergrading and correct the tendency by reestablishing appropriate expectations.

Case Question

How could SW ensure he is not guilty of undergrading SS's interpersonal skills?

PRESENTATION OF THE EVALUATION

Presentation of a final evaluation must be planned appropriately to ensure that the student or resident has the opportunity to fully review the preceptor's scores and written comments. The date, time, and location of the evaluation should have been predetermined. Ideally, you will deliver the evaluation during the final days of the rotation. This is imperative for students because they probably will be moving to another site after the rotation ends and want to know how they performed. For residency evaluations, in particular, it may be difficult to ensure the final evaluations are completed in a timely manner. Residents typically remain onsite longer, creating a sense that timeliness is less important. Delaying this evaluation, however, can seriously diminish the effectiveness of the information provided. Make every effort to complete resident evaluations within 7 days of the end of any learning experience. Final evaluations should be presented in a private setting between the preceptor and the individual student. Plan an adequate amount of time to allow for discussion and addressing the students' questions or concerns. This is an ideal opportunity to provide further suggestions on areas wherein individuals should continue to develop and improve during future rotations.

A preceptor should consider having the student or resident complete a self-assessment using the same evaluation form as the preceptor.[2] Ideally, this would be done before presentation of the preceptor's final evaluation. The student's self-evaluation can then be compared with the preceptor's assessment to stimulate further discussion between the individuals, helping to avoid a one-way conversation. If there is a disagreement between the preceptor's view of the student's performance and the student's self-evaluation, the preceptor can foster self-assessment skills by describing the evidence used to assign the grades, which is the reason why it is important to provide specific comments justifying your scores. You should also be open to the possibility of correcting your evaluation if the student is able to provide sufficient evidence that he or she deserves a higher grade.

Presenting a final evaluation to a student who has not met your expectations, or may even fail a rotation, can be challenging. You may find it difficult to issue a failing grade and, thus, may consider passing the student despite his or her performance, whether it is because you are fond of a student, are afraid of delaying his or her graduation, or are simply averse to confrontation.[3] If a student or resident does not have the knowledge, attitudes, or skills required for the rotation, you must seriously consider failing the individual. In these situations, it is often best to consult with the experiential director of a student's school of pharmacy or a resident's program director for advice. These individuals can review your scoring and comments and provide their perspective. They may be able to provide past information regarding a student's performance on earlier rotations. In many cases, a pattern of less-than-satisfactory performance will be evident, which can provide further support that your assessment is sound. If there are no prior concerns with the student, you may want to consider other reasons for the poor performance. Maybe the student is having a personal issue of which you are unaware? Perhaps the student was unsure of your expectations? Experiential and residency directors can also provide a remediation plan for the student or resident who fails a rotation, including implications related to graduation or successful completion of a residency.

The preceptor should be able to present evidence supporting the student's poor performance. This is when early and frequent documentation of negative performance is essential to providing evidence for the final evaluation. If the preceptor has routinely provided formative feedback throughout the rotation (along with a summative midpoint assessment), the student should not be surprised that a potential failing grade may be on the horizon.

Another challenge is assigning an honors grade to a student. Some of your students will expect to receive this grade for their rotation. These individuals are generally high achievers and may be used to getting good grades. An APPE student may feel that receiving honors on a rotation will help him or her secure a residency. The student may even ask you at the start of a rotation what is required to receive an honors grade. There is mixed opinion on this type of request. Some preceptors may have specific expectations for what constitutes this type of grade and will be open to their students about it. Others look at the student's overall performance to determine if honors will be awarded. As a preceptor, you should be prepared to address such a question from students. When presenting the final evaluation, do not be surprised if your student is disappointed that he or she did not receive honors. How you will respond is largely based on your expectations for such level of achievement.

Quick Tip

Some areas of summative evaluations do not lend themselves to awarding scores higher than "meets expectations." For example, when assessing a learner's professional attire, it may be difficult to determine how the trainee could exceed expectations. For this reason, it is important to identify specific behaviors that would garner higher marks, whenever possible.

A preceptor may also want to use this time to solicit feedback on his or her own performance and the rotation. The end of the rotation is the perfect time to assess your precepting skills, the structure and activities completed during the rotation, and any concerns from your students. Obtaining suggestions for improvements to the rotation can be quite helpful in the future. Students may also be open to sharing an issue that they are reluctant to document on an evaluation form. If a good rapport between the preceptor and student has developed during the rotation, obtaining this feedback should be relatively easy. See Chapter 10 for additional discussion of collecting and using student feedback.

After the final evaluation has been presented, the preceptor should make any final edits and submit it to the college or school of pharmacy or residency director. If there are any concerns with the student's response to the evaluation or the student's overall performance, speak directly to the appropriate individual at the college, school, or residency program to discuss the issue further.

Case Question

If SS truly did not meet expectations for interpersonal communication, how could SW have provided this assessment in a way that would not have come as a surprise during the final evaluation?

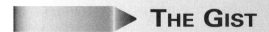

THE GIST

1. Preparing a final evaluation for a pharmacy student or resident requires familiarization of the evaluation criteria, determining one's expectations of student performance, and documentation of student performance throughout the rotation.
2. A preceptor should carefully complete each component of the evaluation, including providing specific written comments to further elaborate on the student's performance.
3. Presentation of a final evaluation should occur just before or on the last day of the rotation in a private setting, with adequate time to address any concerns.
4. Be sure to solicit feedback on the rotation and your own preceptor skills, as well.

SUGGESTED READING

ASHP. The role of your preceptors in evaluating your mastery of educational goals. Chapter 5. In *Resident's Guide to the RLS*, 3rd ed. Bethesda, MD: ASHP; 2006. http://test3-www.ashp.org/DocLibrary/Accreditation/ResidentsGuidetotheRLS.aspx (accessed 8 Apr 2016).

REFERENCES

1. Branch WT, Paranjape A. Feedback and reflection: teaching methods for clinical settings. *Acad Med*. 2002; 77:1185-8.
2. Algiraigri AH. Ten tips for receiving feedback effectively in clinical practice. *Med Educ Online*. 2014; 19:25,141.
3. Dudek NL, Marks MB, Regehr G. Failure to fail: the perspectives of clinical supervisors. *Acad Med*. 2005; 80:S84-7.

◆ APPENDIX 8A ◆

Student APPE Evaluation

Please evaluate the student during the midpoint and final week of the rotation using the following scale for evaluation. A midpoint evaluation is required for any student who is currently performing at an unsatisfactory or needs improvement level. Preceptors are required to provide narrative comments to support Unsatisfactory Performance, Needs Improvement, and Exceeds Expectations scores.

1 Unsatisfactory Performance	2 Needs Improvement	3 Progressing Satisfactorily	4 Exceeds Expectations
Student does not meet requirements. Student is unable to complete basic/ routine tasks despite guidance and prompting.	*Student meets some minimum requirements. Student frequently requires guidance and/or prompting to complete basic or routine tasks.*	*Student consistently meets requirements. Student completes basic and some complex tasks independently with minimal or no guidance and/or prompting.*	*Student exceeds requirements. Student consistently and independently completes all basic and complex tasks going beyond what is required.*

The FINAL rotation grade will be based on student achieving an average of ≥ 2.0 in each section and the average score for all the sections based on the following distribution:

<u>Grading Distribution</u>

Less than 2.5 = Fail

2.5 to 3.5 = Pass

Greater than 3.5 = Pass with Honors

SECTION I: PROFESSIONALISM	Final Week
1. Participates in the process of self-assessment and displays an interest in lifelong learning and continuous professional development	
2. Maintains a professional manner in both appearance and behavior at all times	
3. Demonstrates courtesy and respect toward others and exhibited self-control in all interactions	
4. Maintains confidentiality	
5. Displays cultural sensitivity and tolerance	
6. Arrives on time and prepared for all rotation activities	

Source: Courtesy of Northeast Ohio Medical University College of Pharmacy, Rootstown, OH.

7. Demonstrates appropriate time-management skills and the ability to prioritize	
8. Demonstrates initiative and responsibility for providing patient care and completing assignments	
Comments:	Section Score

SECTION II: COMMUNICATION	Final Week
1. Demonstrates active listening skills and empathy	
2. Effectively communicates both verbally and in writing with patients and other healthcare professionals	
3. Demonstrates the ability to establish effective relationships with other healthcare professionals and patients	
4. Appropriately demonstrates a willingness to form an opinion, express observations, and/or ask questions	
5. Displays effective presentation skills	
6. Demonstrates assertiveness and confidence when making recommendations	
7. Responds to questions in a clear and concise manner with supporting evidence/ rationale via written or verbal communication as appropriate to the situation	
Comments:	Section Score

SECTION III: DRUG/DISEASE KNOWLEDGE	Final Week
1. Demonstrates knowledge of disease states appropriate for this clinical setting	
2. Describes the expected mechanism of action, therapeutic response, adverse effects, and monitoring parameters for a given drug or combination of drugs	
3. Applies physical assessment skills as appropriate to assist in evaluating a patient and his or her medication therapy	
4. Demonstrates knowledge of evidence-based medicine and clinical practice guidelines	
Comments:	Section Score

SECTION IV: APPLICATION	Final Week
Problem Assessment	
1. Uses a systematic problem-solving approach to patient care	
2. Obtains and interprets information from the medical chart, computer system, or patient to assess therapy	
3. Consistently and accurately identifies and prioritizes all medication-related problems	
Plan Development	
1. Designs and evaluates regimens for optimal outcomes, incorporating pharmacokinetic, formulation data, and routes of administration into decision	
2. Adjusts regimens based patient physiologic parameters and response to therapy	
Monitoring Parameters	
1. Creates and implements a monitoring plan to assess the outcomes of drug therapy for a patient	
2. Prospectively measures, records, and tracks a patient's therapeutic response and toxicity to drug therapy	
3. Identifies, assesses, and appropriately reports drug-related problems, adverse events, and toxicities	
4. Assesses patient adherence to medications and risk factors for nonadherence	
Use and Interpretation of Drug Information	
1. Identifies and thoroughly evaluates current literature and effectively applies this information to patient care	
2. Given a drug, health, or operational information question, formulates a timely, efficient, thorough, and effective answer using appropriate sources of information	
3. Provides and appropriately documents references and resources	
Comments:	Section Score

SECTION V: MEDICATION DISTRIBUTION/DISPENSING	Final Week
1. Demonstrates proficiency in processing new and refill prescriptions/medication orders in accordance with regulatory requirements	
2. Accurately selects and prepares appropriate medication for prescription or medication order	
3. Develops a systematic approach for final verification to ensure the five principles of drug delivery: right drug, right patient, right dose, right time, right route	
4. Using the concepts of pharmaceutics and applying best practice guidelines, appropriately compounds products for patient use	
Comments:	Section Score

SECTION VI: ADMINSTRATIVE SKILLS *(to be completed for leadership/management rotations only)*	Final Week
1. Discusses use of management principles (e.g., planning, organizing, directing, and controlling) for simple/individual tasks and complex activities	
2. Discusses and/or participates in resource management related to time, people, finances, and technology/informatics	
3. Discusses and/or participates in quality assurance and/or patient safety activities	
4. Discusses marketing principles and how they are applied	
5. Identifies methods to enhance pharmacy services	
6. Reviews and applies all site-related policies and procedures	
7. Demonstrates an understanding of leadership needs and opportunities in pharmacy practice	
Comments:	Section Score

PRESENTATIONS, JOURNAL CLUBS, ETC.

Provide description/title of presentation and comments on student performance:

PROJECTS, RESEARCH, PUBLICATIONS, ETC.

Provide description of project and comments on student performance:

OVERALL COMMENTS:

LIST AREAS IN NEED OF IMPROVEMENT FOR SUBSQUENT ROTATIONS:

MIDPOINT ROTATION GRADE: _____

FINAL OVERALL ROTATION GRADE: _____

By submitting this evaluation, you confirm that the student has fulfilled all attendance requirements.

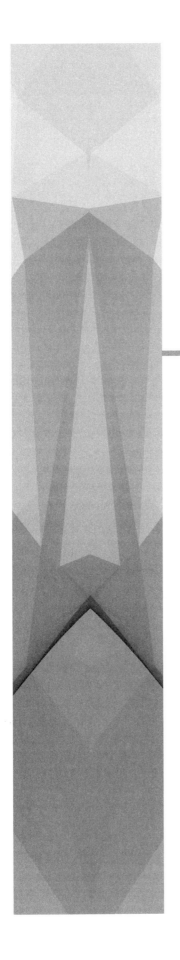

Part III

After the Experience

9. Guidance Beyond the Learning Experience...121
    Stacey R. Schneider

10. Preceptor Assessment and Development.......135
    Jaclyn Boyle

11. Using Learners to Improve Your
    Practice Site 147
    Lukas Everly

Chapter 9

Guidance Beyond the Learning Experience

Stacey R. Schneider

CASE STUDY

JB served as the preceptor for a student at the end of her final year of school. At the final evaluation, she asks JB to be her mentor in guiding her along her career path. When she applies for a residency position, JB is asked to write a letter of recommendation. This is the first recommendation JB has written, and he is afraid his inexperience will hurt his student's chances of obtaining a residency.

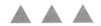

INTRODUCTION

Although many preceptors feel that precepting a learner ends once the final evaluation is completed, preceptors can serve as guides for their students long after the rotation has ended. You will likely serve as a mentor for a number of trainees, leading to fruitful relationships for both of you.

MENTORING

Mentoring is a partnership between a skilled or experienced person (a *mentor*) with a lesser-skilled or experienced person (a *mentee*), with the goal of collaboratively discovering and developing the mentee's abilities and competencies. The mentor helps the mentee reach his or her personal and professional goals by encouraging the mentee's work activities and development through teaching, counseling, supporting, coaching, sponsoring, championing, and identifying networking opportunities. Mentoring is not a forced relationship. As a mentor, you should feel a connection with your mentee and have a true interest in fostering his or her personal and professional growth. The relationship has to be the right fit for both parties for it to grow and be successful.

Building an effective relationship of mutual understanding and trust with your mentee is a critical component of effective mentoring. Mentors can establish rapport with their mentees using effective interpersonal communication skills, actively building trust, and maintaining confidentiality. A mentor who is genuine and nonjudgmental will create an atmosphere for a comfortable relationship. Good verbal and nonverbal communication skills are crucial in the mentoring relationship. Effective communication requires various skills, including active listening, reflecting, summarizing, and using open-ended questions. Active listening requires you to be fully engaged in the task of listening and quieting your own thoughts. This process includes verbally reflecting back what the mentee has just said, ensuring you (the mentor) understand your mentee. During a conversation with your mentee, a summary will help focus the mentee's thoughts and, at times, redirect the conversation, if necessary. Avoid asking closed-ended questions; instead, opt for open-ended questions that encourage your mentee's thoughtful answers in his or her own words.

Although good verbal communication skills are important, a majority of human interaction is nonverbal. Body language, which is a key skill in nonverbal communication, tells those with whom we are communicating a great deal about what we are thinking and feeling. Open body language includes good eye contact, open posture, nodding in affirmation, and a pleasant facial expression. Negative or closed body language includes crossing arms, averting eyes, nodding impatiently, finger pointing, or slumped posture. There may be nonverbal barriers as well, including checking emails or allowing interruptions, which can lead to a lack of sharing of information and sends the message to the mentee of a lack of interest. Therefore, it is essential that the mentor is aware of what he or she is communicating nonverbally as well as what the mentee is communicating nonverbally.

Establishing trust is an essential component in building rapport with a mentee. Along with the communication skills listed above, establishing a trusting dynamic is essential for a productive and positive mentor-mentee relationship. There are numerous ways to establish a trusting relationship, such as sharing appropriate personal experiences from a time when you were mentored or from your clinically relevant experiences. Sharing your own career path often helps the mentee begin to examine his or her own career choices and may lead to new and exciting options not previously considered. Encourage questions of any type, letting the mentee know there are no bad questions. Continually acknowledging the mentee's strengths and accomplishments during the mentoring process is an important step to building self-confidence. Spend some social time with your mentee to get to know them in a nonwork environment. For example, you could schedule a luncheon to learn more about your mentee's personal life and share some things about your own life, within appropriate boundaries. This will also help you understand any cultural differences and further build a personal connection. As with any process, ask for feedback and be open to applying constructive feedback to improve your mentoring skills. Lastly, maintaining confidentiality is a critical component of the mentor-mentee relationship. It will be difficult to establish trust and build rapport if confidentiality is not maintained and there is no respect for privacy.

Quick Tip

The mentoring relationship needs to be an active one. Make regularly scheduled meetings with the mentee part of your workflow.

Four Phases in Mentoring Relationships

There are four different phases to a mentoring relationship[1]:

1. Preparing
2. Negotiating
3. Enabling
4. Closing

Figure 9-1 looks at the different phases and what is involved in each of these phases. It is important to note that a closing for the relationship should be established at the beginning. This may be signified either by a date, such as one year, or a significant mile marker, such as graduation. However, this does not mean the relationship needs to end, it means the relationship needs reevaluation and reflection. It is possible that, through this reflection process, terms are redefined, goals and objectives are updated, and the relationship moves naturally into the next phase. It is also possible that it is time the mentee establishes a new mentor. This should be accomplished after careful reflection by the mentor and mentee with both reaching a conclusion that solidifies the next steps.

Being an Effective Mentor

So how does one go about being an effective mentor? There is a method in the mental health field called *solution-focused therapy*, which is a competency-based model of helping people achieve personal goals.[2] It focuses on strengths and previous successes and not on limitations and shortcomings. The essence of this approach is to explore preferred solutions and what you are already doing to achieve your future goals. The term *solution-focused mentoring* has been patterned to follow the format of this type of therapy.

FIGURE 9-1. PHASES OF A MENTOR-MENTEE RELATIONSHIP

Phases of a Mentor–Mentee Relationship

Negotiating   Enabling

Preparing   Closing

Make the match
and asssess the fit.

Focus on vision and how
to get to the goal.

Plan for career development by
developing a vision, mission,
goals, objectives, and timelines.

Specify a date or mile
marker that will close the
relationship and reflect on
achievements and next steps.

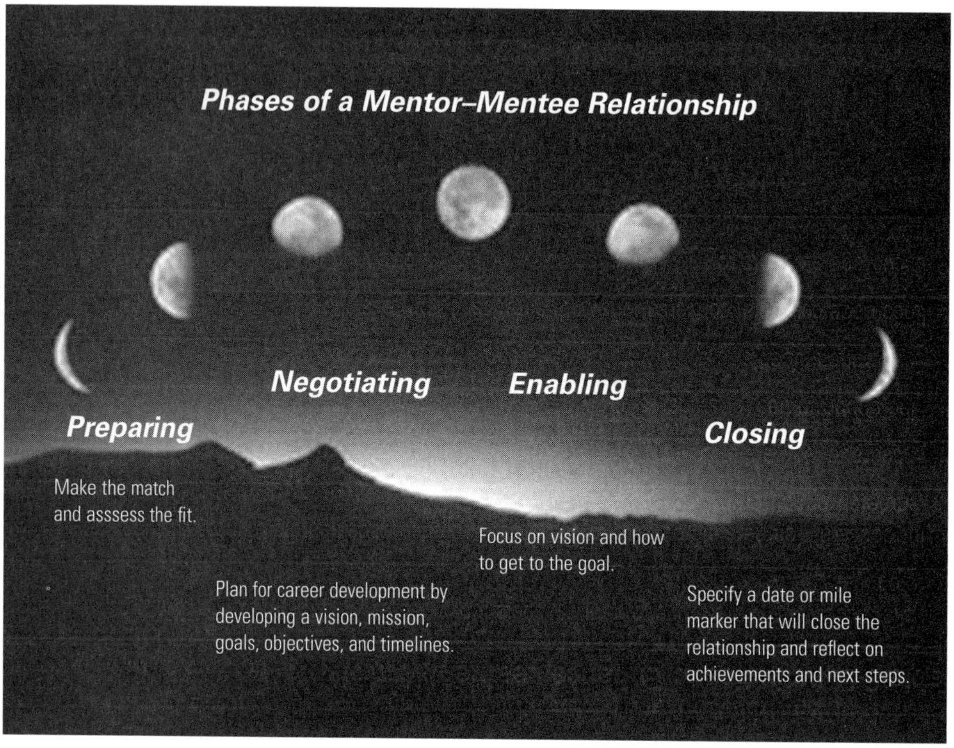

Source: Figure created by Spirit-Fire. Available at: https://www.flickr.com/photos/spirit-fire/6801036620. Courtesy of Common Commons.org.

The premise of the program is to help mentees find their own solutions and determine their individual career paths rather than the mentor recommending solutions or paths that will work for them. The mentor focuses on the mentee's desired future and emphasizes strengths and solutions rather than problems and deficits. The mentor works with the mentee to help identify his or her strengths and how these strengths correlate with job-related preferences. Mentees are encouraged to identify their goals and use their strengths to achieve them. This method draws out the strengths and solutions from within the mentees. In essence, you are asking the mentee to reflect on his or her experiences and identify the most enjoyable aspects to date. Determine how the mentee can get more of these experiences in a career choice and then identify the steps to get to that endpoint. The key to this method is to promote *self-efficacy*, the belief in one's own ability to succeed. Learners with a strong sense of self-efficacy view challenging problems as tasks to master and recover quickly from setbacks. By recognizing strengths and past successes, you will foster confidence and optimism in your mentees. People often fail to recognize their own strengths and successes. A good tool to help your mentees identify their strengths is *StrengthsFinder 2.0*, by Tom Rath.[3] This self-assessment tool will help your mentees identify their top five strengths, which can be a building platform for fostering the career development process discussed in the next section.

Of course, you will not develop a formal mentoring relationship with all of your students or residents. However, there are brief episodes, referred to as *mentoring moments*, which are very different from the formal mentoring relationship but are also important. This type of mentoring is situational and can occur each day as you precept your learners and is likely occurring even if you are unaware of it. They are the brief teaching and learning moments we have on a daily basis that go beyond teaching basic knowledge and skills. Whether you are acting in a formal or informal mentoring situation, becoming an effective mentor takes time and practice. The benefit of having both a formal mentor-mentee relationship and acting to facilitate mentoring moments during your rotation will all serve as valuable tools to build highly effective healthcare practitioners.

Case Question

JB's student would like to meet regularly to discuss career development and review her progress toward achieving her career goals. Is this relationship shaping up to be formal mentor-mentee relationship or does it fall into the realm of informal mentoring situations?

CAREER DEVELOPMENT

One of the key aspects and benefits of a mentoring relationship is career development. This is the lifelong process of combining learning, work, leisure, and transitions to move toward a personally determined future. It takes active work to set goals, make decisions, and gather information so you make the best choice possible about your future. To do this, one must be skilled at self-assessment and reflecting on experiences and feelings related to his or her professional goals. This is a holistic view of life because it relates to not only our professional goals but also our personal values, personalities, and interests. One must take into account the ever-changing relationships, needs, and desires both at work and in personal life. Amazingly enough, these can all be congruent and, in a best-case scenario, will satisfy each other.

It can be an overwhelming process to start, so it is best to begin with self-assessment. Understanding who you are is critical to finding the correct career path. Ask your mentees to begin by stating their skills or strengths. Perhaps this is a time to refer back to the StrengthsFinder exercise mentioned earlier and reflect on those strengths. Keep in mind, just because you have a particular skill set or strength does not mean you enjoy doing it. Ask your mentees to think about what excites them. You may ask, "What interests you enough that when you are doing it you lose track of time?"

Next, identify values. Before setting goals, you need to decide what is important to you (e.g., what your values are). *Values* are a set of standards that determine your attitudes, choices, and actions. They are the qualities and principles that guide you as you set priorities in your career and life. They are highly personal and define what is purposeful and meaningful to you. Values may change in response to life circumstances, but they are generally enduring and will guide you in making career decisions. Conflict between the work we do and the work we value is often at the root of our decisions to change careers. Defining your values will ensure that your career starts off on the right path.

As a mentor, you can be a critical factor in guiding your mentees in defining their values. Asking your mentees some key questions can help facilitate this process. Refer to Table 9-1 for questions and an abbreviated list of values. Have your mentees keep a list of their important values to refer back to during this process. If you help your mentees identify what they believe in, chances are they will be on the correct career paths.

The final step is setting short- and long-term goals. Goals should be specific, measurable, attainable, relevant, and timely. Once goals are determined, action should be taken to help reach those goals. Because this is a continual process, your mentees will need to reassess how this process is going. This would be a great time as a mentor to do some reflecting with your mentees. There will be times when goals may change a bit if the mentees find something that is a better fit. That's what the experiential and residency process is all about! Encourage them to use the information they have collected as guides toward their ultimate decisions.

I have had students on my rotation do a fun (they may tell you excruciating) exercise to help them define their career paths. Although a time-consuming and difficult process, all of them agreed it was extremely worthwhile and helped them to grow, not only professionally but personally, as well. Along with the above suggestions of defining values, and setting short- and long-term goals, the students were asked to think of their perfect day at work. They were encouraged to write in detail what that perfect day would look like. We also did an exercise that entailed what they wanted to be remembered for. If someone were writing your eulogy, what would they say about you? Yes, this seems a little morbid, but stick with me! I encouraged them to consider what they wanted their life to look like and what they wanted to accomplish. I asked them to pretend that rather than graduating, starting a career, and moving on toward the rest of their lives, they were at the end of it. How would people remember them, as both a person and a professional? The point of this exercise is to think about how they wanted to be remembered by family, friends, and colleagues and then let this shape their chosen path. I now have a treasured collection as to what I refer to as *Mission Statements*. See Box 9-1 for a sample mission statement.

Table 9-1. Revealing Values in Career Development

Question	Related Values
♦ What motivates you to love your job each day?	Achievement, power, prestige, making an impact
♦ What work conditions are optimal for you to perform your best work?	Flexibility, excitement, predictability, geographic location
♦ What makes your work activities satisfying and will engage your interests on a regular basis?	Leading, challenging, learning, social activism
♦ What types of interactions with your colleagues are most important to you?	Collaboration, autonomy, diversity, humor

---

Box 9-1. Sample Mission Statement

Mission

To live honestly, compassionately, and fully each day. To make a positive impact, even in a small way, in someone's life each day. To always serve others first.

Vision

To improve the health and well-being of others through education, compassion, and mentoring. To serve others while working toward shared goals of making the world a better place. To give back, inspire, and lead others in a positive way. To act with integrity and honesty in working on established relationships and building new ones.

Values

- Honesty
- Integrity
- Humility
- Compassion
- Leadership
- Positivity

Goals

Short-Term Goals

- To develop leadership skills to advance the profession of pharmacy.
- To mentor students in the career development process and provide new opportunities for their growth.
- To develop my teaching style and establish new methods of pedagogy that incorporate innovative teaching methods.
- To remain and become more involved in organizational work to collaboratively move pharmacy forward.
- To seek professional development opportunities that will lead to future leadership roles.
- To maintain and develop relationships with family, friends, colleagues, students, and the community.

Long-Term Goals

- To mentor and inspire others to make a positive change in the world.
- To advance the profession of pharmacy through organization work and advocacy involvement.
- To pursue job opportunities that will allow me to grow professionally and personally.
- To give back to my community through service, philanthropy, and volunteerism.

(continued)

BOX 9-1. SAMPLE MISSION STATEMENT (CONTINUED)

How Do You Wish to Be Remembered?

♦ She was both a teacher and a learner.
♦ She always worked to benefit others.
♦ She was a servant leader who was humble and modest in her leadership style.
♦ She maintained a well-balanced life both personally and professionally.
♦ She sought new opportunities.
♦ She lived each day to the fullest.
♦ She was excited by change.
♦ She was grateful.
♦ She left a legacy of living life with love and positivity.

My Ideal Day

My ideal day starts and ends in prayer. I am thankful for the opportunity to have the chance to live another day. It starts and ends with telling my husband how much I love him and thanking him for his dedication and support. Sprinkled in my day is time connecting with friends, family, and colleagues trying to touch their lives in positive ways.

I will have creative and innovative work taking care of patients or teaching and learning with others how best to take care of patients. I will make time to exercise and have a healthy diet all while maintaining time for myself.

Each day will be an opportunity to read and seek new opportunities to learn.

I will listen to a short snippet of news to keep up with what's going on outside of my world. At the end of the day I am assured I attempted to live each day to the fullest and maximized the time I have.

Case Question

JB is meeting with his student to discuss her newly written mission statement. How can this document be used to help his mentee develop her career?

Quick Tip

Defining your own mission statement and discussing it with your learners can help them identify steps to work through to aid them in their own career development.

WRITING LETTERS OF RECOMMENDATION

You may be asked to write letters of recommendations for your students or residents. There are a few things to consider before writing a letter of recommendation. First, consider if you are able to write a positive letter of recommendation. If not, invite the student for an honest conversation about how you feel and leave it open to the student to decide if they would like you to write the letter. A negative or even a neutral recommendation letter may seriously harm a student's ability to be accepted into a residency or job. Second, consider if you know enough about the student to write a letter that best speaks to their abilities. Depending on your role as a preceptor, you may not have spent enough time with the student. Therefore, it may be wise to say "no" and encourage the student to ask someone who spent more time during a rotation seeing the student perform. The student should have the person most familiar with their abilities write the letter so the writer can speak adequately to their skills, knowledge, and maturity.

Alternatively, you may meet with the student to discuss his or her career goals and get the additional information necessary to write an appropriate letter. Asking why the student has chosen this position will help you tailor your recommendation letters. Consider discussing why the student has chosen you to write a recommendation. It might be because he or she particularly enjoyed your rotation or did very good work for you, or simply because a recommendation is needed from a preceptor with your experience and background. Having this conversation will bring to mind specific preceptor-student interactions that will help you to avoid generalizations in your letter. Last, consider your workload and determine if you will have adequate time to write a meaningful letter. It can be quite a time commitment to write letters of recommendation, and you should always take into account your schedule as well as the deadline the student has provided.

The following tips should help you prepare for the writing stage:

♦ Consider requesting adequate material from students to ensure you will give detailed descriptions of their achievements, skills, knowledge, and future career goals. You may ask for the student's curriculum vitae, transcripts, projects, or assignments from other rotations.

♦ Collect information such as a description of the position that is being applied for, any required forms, the recipient of the letter, and address for forwarding. Always address the recommendation letter to the appropriate person. "To Whom It May Concern" is a last resort.

♦ Print your recommendation letter out on the letterhead that represents your site, reinforcing your professionalism and authority.

All of these tips will help to ensure your letter appears professional.

The recommendation letter usually consists of four major parts: your relationship with the student, the student's performance, the student's characteristics, and summary of accomplishments and qualities. The first section usually states your relationship with the student, how long you have known them, and in what context. You may choose to include a description of the practice setting and highlight the student's responsibilities. The second section should discuss the student's performance on your rotation. This section should be specific and detailed. List those things that the student did exceptionally well while on rotation. Important skills to consider would be communication, autonomy, knowledge base, critical thinking, and teamwork skills. Give details as to how the student displayed these skills. Merely listing positive attributes with no explanations may appear insincere or inaccurate. The third section typically addresses a student's characteristics. Even though you are discussing intangibles in this section, you should avoid exaggerated statements and generalizations. Choosing to say, "She is a good mentor to other students" is inadequate. Provide concrete examples of what you mean when you say the student is a good mentor, mentioning specific interactions you witnessed. The final section is your chance to summarize the student's qualities or accomplishments that you wish to emphasize such as awards, leadership roles, or an excellent academic record. You should summarize the enthusiasm you have for the student to be a good candidate for the position and end with an invitation to contact you if further information is requested.

Sometimes you will be required to write about the applicant's weaknesses or areas for improvement. If that is the case, provide thoughtful criticism and ways in which you saw the student improving during the rotation. You could also tie criticism of the student to your own ethics. For example, you might state that as a recommender you feel obligated to give a balanced assessment of your student in contrast to the typical recommendation letter that offers biased praise. Some may read a letter that is entirely full of over-the-top praise with skepticism. Therefore, it may be beneficial to the student to provide your assessment of areas in need of improvement. Demonstrating that the student shows an active interest in improving themselves is a critical skill for a professional and will shed a positive light on the student.

Finally, keep in mind that the letter of recommendation should not merely repeat what is listed on the student's resume. Keep your letter focused and personal to enhance the sincerity of your praise. Very short letters can send a negative message and very long letters are a chore to read. A good guide is to keep your letter between one to two pages in length. Before final submission, proofread your letter and, if available, have a colleague read it, as well, especially if you are not a seasoned writer.

Box 9-2 contains a sample letter of recommendation.

NETWORKING FOR YOU AND YOUR LEARNER

Most of us were not taught how to network as part of our pharmacy curriculum. To impart this important skill to our students, we must first have mastered the skill as a preceptor. *Networking* is defined as the process of meeting people, either through a contact that you initiate or through an introduction by a third party. It is not something that we are born knowing how to do; it is more of a learned skill. At our core, we are human beings who want to connect with other human beings. Networking is about building relationships—a two-way street of helpful relationships. Think about networking in a different light for a moment. Each day we come across questions and have problems to solve. How do we get the answers? We may search the Internet for the answer, but there are certain people we go to regularly for their ability to provide good recommendations. Networking is about getting answers to our questions from people we know and respect. Modeling successful people with your shared goals and values is a proven way to improve your own performance. By surrounding yourself with colleagues you want to emulate, their attitudes, habits, and associations will rub off. A good network will surround you with people you admire and respect and will likely have a profound impact on your life and work.

BOX 9-2. SAMPLE LETTER OF RECOMMENDATION

November 30, 2016

Leslie Smith, PharmD
Residency Program Director
General Health System
Department of Pharmacy
500 School Street
Pasadena, Ohio 00000

Dear Dr. Smith,

This letter is in support of Joan Student's application for the PGY1 residency at the General Health System Department of Pharmacy. I have known Joan since she began her education at our college four years ago. She recently spent a month with me on rotation at my community practice site. This site is an ambulatory care clinic where I work with physicians to ensure patients have optimal medication regimens, counseling, and assessment of adherence issues. During this rotation, Joan worked with an interprofessional team to facilitate patient care. Her responsibilities included medication therapy management visits, consulting patients in a diabetes and lipids clinic, and teaching medical residents during grand rounds. She not only possesses a strong background of clinical knowledge but also uses critical thinking that translates into practical patient care in a real-life setting. Comments from the interprofessional team stated that she was a viable part of the team due to her readiness to answer drug information questions and her on-the-spot teaching about medications to her colleagues. The site has numerous responsibilities and requires efficient time management skills and an ability to practice autonomously. Joan successfully mastered these skills and was timely with all projects including case presentations, journal clubs, and occasional precepting of other students.

Coming from such a diverse background is one of Joan's many strengths. All of the challenges she has faced in her lifetime have given her the insight to understand and empathize with patients. She was able to convey a level of sincerity to make patients feel comfortable with her and enable her to form a professional trusting relationship with them. This skill was beyond what I see most of my students able to do. I was also impressed with her maturity and insight in the areas where she needed improvement. She was continually eager for feedback and strived to improve with each learning experience. We worked to develop her assertive skills, and I believe with time and confidence Joan will establish a comfortable level of assertiveness. She is determined to achieve the goals she has set for herself and works diligently each day to make sure she is on the correct path. There were times when she overwhelmed me with her continuous enthusiasm for the profession and her skills to help her patients. She is clearly passionate about being a pharmacist and with dedicated perseverance will achieve her goals.

Joan has truly dedicated herself to the profession as is evident in her many leadership positions in student organizations. She has also dedicated her time to service in the community by volunteering to assist in numerous activities. It is clear she values the well-being of her community and will work to help those in need. I believe all of these qualities will make her an asset to the profession of pharmacy.

In summary, Joan would be an excellent candidate for your residency program, and I urge you to give her your highest consideration. Please feel free to contact me with any additional questions.

Sincerely,

JB, PharmD

Networking, like its name implies, is work. It can be an easy skill to learn for extroverts, but is especially painful if you are an introvert. Shyness can be an insurmountable roadblock to networking for many professionals. However, understanding how to network effectively is the key to success. It is never about making a direct request. Instead, it is about chatting one-on-one with someone you know (or someone who was suggested you get to know) about common interests and how you might help them. The key is to create a basic script and practice it. This will allow you to get the conversation started and overcome your natural hesitancy to talk about yourself. To break the ice with a new contact, ask about his or her family, job, interests, or perhaps something as simple as the latest book he or she has read. If you are searching for a new job opportunity, you could launch into something like, "I was looking forward to meeting you because I am eager to find new opportunities that challenge my interests and speak to my passion in pharmacy. Would you happen to know any opportunities that may be available for me to pursue?" This script can be revised in many ways and provides a nonthreatening means to turn casual conversation into a great source of leads or contacts. The key to becoming comfortable and confident in your networking skills is continual practice.

If you are one of those people who hate to network and view it as phony or pretentious, perhaps you are doing it all wrong. Networking is not about building a giant list of contacts or seeing who can pass out the most business cards. This leads to an artificial contact list. Instead, networking means building mutually beneficial relationships.

There are some common mistakes people make when trying to network.

- *First, avoid the misconception that networking should be done only when you need a job.* Building a network takes time, and when you are in a crisis situation you will be very disappointed with your network if you have not invested time in it. Instead, set aside time on a regular basis to stay in touch with past colleagues and to meet new people so your network will be there when you need it.
- *Do not limit your networking activity to local, regional, or national professional meetings.* Although these meetings are critical to your networking opportunities, be aware that networking can occur at any place and at any time. All you need to do is be open to the possibilities of meeting someone new.
- *Follow up with new contacts.* If you have been busy building your network but have not followed up, it is easy for people to forget you. It is your responsibility to stay in touch with those in your network. Share information with them, offer to be of assistance, or invite them to join you at an event. Put a date on your calendar each month to carve time out for staying in contact with your network.
- *A common misconception is that networking is only about helping oneself.* However, networking is also about helping others. Show genuine interest in other people's passions, continue to ask them questions, and listen for opportunities to offer help or make a new connection. If you are not taking an interest in your colleagues' lives, they will likely see through your intentions and could get the feeling that you are not genuinely interested in them.
- *Learn everything you can about a new contact before your meeting.* You may consider preparing questions to help stimulate the conversation. Given the opportunity, most people love to talk about themselves. Not being prepared is bound to have a negative impact on your meeting.

♦ *Be genuine and likeable.* Remember, you get only one chance to make a positive first impression—and first impressions are the most lasting.

Social media is a great way to expand your network and meet people you would never have met otherwise. Some social media tools include LinkedIn, Facebook, and Twitter. Through LinkedIn you can congratulate a colleague on a new position, post your connection status updates on yourself, and view changes to your other colleagues updates. You can also endorse someone else's talents which may be helpful if they are looking for new connections, follow group discussions, and add your feedback to the conversation. Facebook and Twitter allow you to follow other individuals and identify friends of friends that could be added to your network. The key to social media is to engage in it on a regular basis. This means setting aside time in your calendar. Some recommend engaging in social media on a daily basis, but you must do what works for you.

Once you have developed your own networking skills, you can serve as a valuable asset for your residents and students. Plug your trainees into your network to allow them to practice their own networking skills and give them a head start toward building a network of their own. Networking for information about career opportunities may be crucial to helping them secure a position that suits them. Also, teaching them the skills of effective networking will prove to be a valuable resource as they transition through their careers. Model the skills of networking for your learners. For various activities to jump-start your learner's networking skills refer to Table 9-2. Teaching your students how to network and broaden their professional horizons will provide them with valuable skills for continual career development.

Case Question

JB plans to participate in a local pharmacy organization. His student is also interested in attending. How could JB use this pharmacy organization as a means to develop his student's network?

Table 9-2. Activities to Enhance Learner Networking

♦ Take students to professional meetings, social activities at your site, or dinners with colleagues to emulate networking skills.

♦ Introduce all learners at your site to one other and encourage sharing of interests (include learners from different professions).

♦ Encourage learners to share the results of a project to others who may be interested.

♦ Find opportunities for students to give talks at local, state, or regional levels.

♦ Encourage students to bond with their peers, not just dignitaries in the field.

♦ Encourage continual conversations with established professionals.

♦ Encourage students to ask a question at every lecture attended to gain confidence speaking in front of others.

> ## THE GIST
>
> 1. The key to a successful mentoring relationship includes creating a trusting relationship; defining roles and responsibilities; and establishing goals, open communication, and collaboration.
> 2. The key to writing a letter of recommendation that is genuine, original, polished, and professional is to make sure you have adequately prepared for the process by gathering all pertinent information about the learner.
> 3. Networking keeps you sharp, current, and in touch with the profession and will keep a career from stagnating. It is important to not only develop your trainees' clinical skills but to also show them how to build and maintain their professional networks.

SUGGESTED READING

Jong ED. Solution focused mentoring: 5 Steps to bring out the best in your mentee and yourself. http://bookboon.com/en/solution-focused-mentoring-ebook (accessed 15 Oct 2016).

Rath T. *StrengthsFinder 2.0*. New York: Gallup Press; 2007.

REFERENCES

1. Zachary LJ. *The Mentor's Guide: Facilitating Effective Learning Relationships*. 2nd ed. San Francisco: Jossey-Bass; 2011.
2. Greenberg G, Ganshorn K, Danelkiwich AD. Solution-focused therapy. Counseling model for busy family physicians. *Can Fam Physician*. 2001; 47:2289-95.
3. Rath T. *StrengthsFinder 2.0*. New York: Gallup Press; 2007.

Chapter 10

Preceptor Assessment and Development

Jaclyn Boyle

CASE STUDY

TR is a new preceptor starting ambulatory services at a physician-based outpatient clinic. He is taking one resident on an elective rotation. TR designated the rotation as a patient care experience because he believed services would be up and running by the start of the rotation. As the rotation is approaching, he has not yet established a practice with the primary care physician in the clinic and is nervous about the quality of the rotation.

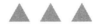

INTRODUCTION

This chapter serves as an introduction to preceptor assessment and development. While not intended to be an all-inclusive guide, it will help you think critically about formal and informal learner feedback opportunities, assessment of precepting abilities, and developing strategies for continuous professional development related to precepting learners. Why are the aforementioned considerations essential to effective precepting? Without reflection and thoughtful application of feedback from learners, your precepting abilities may become stagnant or ineffective. Preceptors owe it to their learners to be continuously improving because learners are asked to continuously improve, as well.

GATHERING LEARNER FEEDBACK

How often are we asking our learners for feedback about our precepting abilities? Gathering learner feedback is essential to improve learning experiences and to ensure you understand how your learners feel about the learning experience. Learner feedback can be gathered in many ways and can be used to continuously improve your learning experience. Feedback should be intentionally built into the learning experience for both the learner and the preceptor. Without a reciprocation of feedback on a regular basis, learners may feel that their opinion is not valued or welcome.

Informal Feedback

Informal feedback can be given at any time and in a variety of formats. Consider setting up regular meetings with your learners on a daily or weekly basis. You can easily couple your formative evaluation of learners with an opportunity to gather feedback on your precepting style and the rotation.

Some questions you should consider asking are:

◆ How do you feel this learning experience is going?
◆ What can I do to improve your learning experience?
◆ Is there anything you wish you could learn about that you haven't had a chance to experience?

Remember, learners may be hesitant to give feedback to you as a preceptor because they may feel intimidated by this encounter. Consider providing one or more open invitations to talk throughout the experience to ensure feedback is a routine part of your activities. Also, encourage your learners that their feedback is not only helpful from your perspective, but also their feedback will help future learners. Taking notes during meetings with your learners can be helpful in monitoring your progress with them. Additionally, such notes can help with self-reflection of your teaching abilities and how to adapt to different types of learners.

Summative Preceptor Evaluations

Like summative evaluations of learners, summative evaluations of preceptors are formal, comprehensive scheduled evaluations that usually take place at the midpoint and final evaluation. Although these evaluations are typically required for each rotation, you may need to exert some effort to gain actionable evaluations (many students fall into the habit of providing only a few comments on evaluation forms). Prompting your learners with the aforementioned reasons to provide both positive reinforcement and constructive criticism of your precepting prior to the summative evaluation may allow the learners to provide honest and open feedback. Often, learners may be hesitant to be completely open and honest. They may think that providing a negative evaluation of their preceptor may result in a lower grade. Reinforcing that evaluations are simply completed to improve the learning experience can be one way to alleviate such fears. Discuss encouraging students to provide examples of how they would change aspects of the rotation they did not like. This allows them to feel comfortable providing potentially negative feedback in a more constructive, solution-based manner.

Quick Tip

Encourage learners to complete evaluations in a timely manner. According to the ASHP residency standard, residents must complete and discuss an evaluation of each learning experience within 7 days of the due date.[1] When evaluations occur directly after the learning experience has ended, recall bias can be minimized and suggestions for improvement can be implemented in time to benefit the next group of learners.

Exit Interviews

Another way to collect your learner's feedback is to conduct an exit interview. The exit interview is a scheduled, sit-down discussion of a learning experience and is often used for experiences that are more longitudinal in nature (rotations spanning multiple months or interviews conducted at the end of the residency year).

Some questions that may be asked during the exit interview include:

- What is your perception of the culture of the organization?
- What is your perception of the pharmacy department?
- How did you feel about your interactions with the pharmacy team during your learning experience?
- How can we improve our learning experience?
- What were strengths of the learning experience?
- What were the most difficult aspects of this learning experience?
- How did this rotation stack up against similar rotations completed by your peers?
- What advice would you give to incoming learners?
- What is one thing you would change for future learners?
- What did your preceptor(s) do that helped you learn?
- What did your preceptor(s) do that hindered your learning?
- What did you gain from this rotation?
- How did this experience impact your learning?

Valuable information can be collected via the exit interview, however, a fair amount of miscellaneous information may also be collected. As such, information collected from the exit interview about the current experience as well as proposed changes for future learners' experiences should be collated to identify trends across multiple learners. One-time issues or isolated events may not trigger a significant change in the learning experience structure or in a preceptor's teaching style. However, if themes emerge, the information may be used to create an action plan to ensure continuous quality improvement of the learning experience. These changes should only occur as long as such feedback is still applicable to the current practice site. A documented and structured exit interview form may help standardize this process. Preceptors should review their exit interview questions on a regular basis to ensure they are effectively collecting data that will benefit the program and future learners.

Postcompletion Surveys

Another avenue for gathering learner feedback could be the creation of surveys to be administered to trainees after they complete the rotation. This survey can be done anonymously or with identifiable information. Anonymous surveys may allow the learners to provide more open and honest feedback to the preceptor regarding concerns or the rotation's shortcomings.

Examples of postcompletion survey questions that could gather more information about the site or the specific rotation are:

◆ How did you feel this site contributed to your overall learning/development?
◆ What could be improved about this site/rotation?
◆ How did you feel about the resources provided to you throughout the rotation?
◆ Discuss aspects of the rotation/site that you found to be great learning experiences.
◆ Discuss aspects of the rotation/site that you found less desirable as a learning experience.
◆ Would you recommend this site/rotation to another learner? Why?
◆ What do you wish you would have known before starting your experience at this site?
◆ Is there any other important information you hope to contribute back to the site/rotation?
◆ Following completion of this rotation, how do you think your future practice will be impacted?

Case Question

At the end of the rotation, TR sits down with the resident to determine how he felt about the month-long experience. Realizing that the rotation may not have lived up to the resident's expectations, TR is somewhat hesitant to hear his feedback. Given this scenario, what are some important questions TR might ask the resident to improve the rotation in the future?

PRECEPTOR SELF-ASSESSMENT

Although learner feedback is vital to assessing a learning experience, it is also important for preceptors to set aside time for self-reflection and self-evaluation. Depending on the time frame, you may consider performing a self-evaluation at the end of every learning experience (or at some regular interval) to determine how to continuously develop professionally in the precepting arena. If self-assessment is not a routine occurrence or you are unsure of where to begin, suggestions and guidance are outlined below.

For those precepting pharmacy residents, ASHP has published requirements of qualified preceptors within their residency standard documents. These criteria are an excellent starting point as you begin to evaluate your own preceptor qualifications.

To qualify as a preceptor under ASHP standards, preceptors must meet the following expected requirements[2]:

1. Demonstrate the ability to precept residents' learning experiences by use of clinical teaching roles (i.e., instructing, modeling, coaching, facilitating) at the level required by the residents
2. Demonstrate the ability to assess residents' performance
3. Possess recognition in the area of pharmacy practice for which they serve as preceptors
4. Possess an established, active practice in the area for which they serve as preceptor
5. Maintain continuity of practice during the time of residents' learning experiences
6. Demonstrate ongoing professionalism, including a personal commitment to advancing the profession

Based on the above criteria, you may consider conducting an individualized SWOT (strengths. weaknesses, opportunities, threats) analysis of your own precepting abilities. Following this SWOT analysis, preceptors may take this information and begin to form strategic SMART (specific, measureable, attainable, relevant, time-bound) goals related to their own preceptor development. Gaps in your qualifications and the residency standard can be identified through this process, leading to the creation of a preceptor development plan to remedy any deficiencies. If you are precepting student pharmacists or other student learners, this exercise may be helpful during a discussion with your supervisor or the experiential director at an affiliated college or school of pharmacy. See Table 10-1 for a SWOT analysis template.

Case Question

TR completes a SWOT analysis after his rotation with his first resident. After reviewing his SWOT analysis, he would like to develop three SMART goals related to precepting that can be accomplished before his next rotation begins. Develop a SMART goal for each of the following rotation improvements:

- *Standardizing activities that every learner will complete on the rotation*
- *Attending preceptor development training*
- *Providing formative feedback regularly to residents*

For preceptors of student pharmacists, the Accreditation Council for Pharmacy Education requires each college or school of pharmacy to establish criteria for preceptor recruitment, orientation, performance, and evaluation. Therefore, preceptors should familiarize themselves with the college's or school's preceptor criteria, as well as associated evaluation materials.[4] Additionally, the American College of Clinical Pharmacy has published a list of recommendations for preceptors who teach student pharmacists based on experience type.[5]

Table 10-1. SWOT Analysis Template	
Strengths	**Weaknesses**
What are the key qualities that I possess that contribute to successful precepting? In what settings do I feel most comfortable teaching?	What are some areas of precepting that I should focus on improving/receiving continuous professional development in? What can I do differently to help my students'/residents' learning process?
Opportunities	**Threats**
What opportunities exist at my site that my learners might benefit from being involved/incorporated? Where can I find continuous professional development to expand/improve my precepting abilities?	What resources do I lack to improve as a preceptor? What barriers exist? What site factors may hinder or negatively impact learning experiences?

Source: Adapted from ASHP Accreditation Standard for Postgraduate Year One (PGY1) Pharmacy Residency Programs. Used with permission ©ASHP, Bethesda, MD.

To ensure that precepting is a continuously improving process, residency programs and sites with student learners should consider developing standardized plans for preceptor assessment and development. ASHP has published one example of a Preceptor Development Plan (see Table 10-2).[6]

Quick Tip

Residency programs and schools of pharmacy may consider assessing preceptor development by reviewing preceptor self-assessments, the quality and content of documented learner feedback, learner evaluations of the preceptor, or by conducting a focus group of previous trainees.

Table 10-2. Preceptor Development Plan	
Group Development	**Preceptor-Specific Development/ Action Plans (As Needed)**
New preceptor workshop (required) ♦ Learning experience activities ♦ Four preceptor teaching roles ♦ Criteria-based feedback ♦ Evaluation strategies ♦ Other (identified from assessment)	Direct feedback to preceptors (RPD, pharmacy administration)
Monthly Topic Discussions at RAC or staff meetings[a]	Reading and computer-based training
Quarterly Lunch 'n' Learn or dinner programs	Mentoring program
Workshops/conferences/courses	Workshops/conferences/courses

[a]Topics decided by annual preceptor needs assessments.
RAC = residency advisory committee, RPD = residency program director.
Source: Adapted from ASHP's Residency Program Design and Conduct (RPDC) Workshops. Used with permission ©ASHP, Bethesda, MD.

Professional Development and Goal Setting

Precepting is a skill that requires continuous professional development over time. Setting aside time for self-reflection and goal setting is essential for all aspects of your professional life including practice skills, service, and teaching. There may be a particular time of the week that can be set aside for self-reflection and goal setting as it relates to various aspects of your responsibilities. Making notes to yourself based on learner feedback and evaluating how your goals and values line up with teaching responsibilities can help align your learning experiences with your overall professional goals. It may be reasonable to reflect on experiences at the end of each week, while thoughts are fresh in your mind.

In self-reflection, you should consider the following questions to help guide your reflecting process:

♦ What do I enjoy most about precepting?
♦ What do I find most challenging about precepting?
♦ Where do I feel I excel in my precepting abilities?
♦ Where do I feel I could improve in my precepting abilities?
♦ What environmental factors (either positively or negatively) impact my precepting abilities?
♦ What steps can I take in the next (week, month, year) to improve my precepting abilities?
♦ What feedback have I received from my learners?
♦ What feedback have I received from my colleagues and superiors?

To improve your existing precepting skills, you should consider developing a plan and identifying means to further develop those skills. Such continuous development will not only contribute to your professional development, but will also result in beneficial effects for your practice site and learners. Additionally, discussing precepting topics and skills with other preceptors can foster new ideas and methods to sharpen existing skills. Consider offering to develop continuing education or faculty development sessions related to precepting topics, as this can be a great way to not only learn about precepting, but to teach it to your colleagues, as well.

Resources to Aid Developing Your Skills

There are many resources available to aid in the development of precepting skills. To help you develop your own preceptor development plan, many tools and resources can be found at: http://www.ashp.org/menu/PracticePolicy/ResourceCenters/Residency-Resource-Center/Program-Self-Assessment. One additional consideration would be to substitute the new ASHP Preceptor eligibility and qualifications, as well.[2] Other venues to acquire preceptor development include[7]:

♦ Attending professional organization meetings
♦ Contributing to or reviewing publications related to precepting
♦ Seeking out online training:
  ▪ www.pharmacistsletter.com
  ▪ www.ashp.org/accreditation
  ▪ www.ashp.org/preceptorskills
  ▪ www.aacp.org/career/educationscholar

♦ Completing a self-assessment rubric such as the sample from ASHP (see Table 10-3)

Additional Suggestions for Developing Precepting Skills

Another way to develop precepting skills is by contributing to scholarly activity related to precepting and preceptor development, including teaching opportunities and scholarly activities (newsletters, research, publications, etc.) that focus on precepting. You may consider collaborating with colleagues who are interested in this topic and developing methods to easily integrate scholarship as a regular part of your daily responsibilities. Consider contributing to a department or site newsletter. If unavailable, perhaps you can take the lead on the implementation of a newsletter for your site. Many staff members and learners enjoy contributing to an informal publication such as a newsletter, disseminating the work of content production across multiple preceptors. Another consideration would be to become a peer reviewer for a journal of interest. This will not only allow you to provide service to the profession, but may be helpful in improving your writing skills, as well.

Asking for Feedback from Colleagues and Superiors

Last, you may consider seeking an outsider's perspective of your precepting skills from colleagues, residency directors, or the residency advisory committee. If regular feedback is not already a part of your evaluation procedures, you should consider seeking feedback from individuals who have had the opportunity to witness your precepting skills. Ideally, this feedback session would be scheduled in a private manner to ensure an open dialogue and allow confidential information to be discussed. One consideration for residency programs is to schedule preceptor development meetings throughout the year to ensure a continuous quality improvement process for precepting. For those precept-

Table 10-3. ASHP Preceptor Self-Assessment	
1. How do you rate your performance as a pharmacy practice role model for residents?	Poor Superb 1 2 3 4 5
2. How do you rate your performance of providing regular formative and summative feedback to residents in a timely manner?	Poor Superb 1 2 3 4 5
3. Do you make yourself available for resident interaction on a regular basis?	Never Always 1 2 3 4 5
4. Do you arrange necessary opportunities to allow residents to complete all learning objectives listed in your rotation?	Never Always 1 2 3 4 5
5. How well do you display enthusiasm for teaching?	Poor Superb 1 2 3 4 5
6. How well do you answer questions clearly and give clear explanations to the resident?	Poor Superb 1 2 3 4 5
7. Do you ask the residents questions that cause self-directed learning?	Never Always 1 2 3 4 5
8. How well do you perform the four preceptor roles of direct instruction, modeling, coaching, and facilitating?	Poor Superb 1 2 3 4 5
9. How do you display interest in the resident?	

Source: http://www.ashp.org/DocLibrary/Accreditation/Residency-Learning-System/RTP-Preceptor-Self-Assessment-Example.aspx.

ing introductory pharmacy practice experience (IPPE) or advanced pharmacy practice experience (APPE) students, requesting feedback from the college or school of pharmacy can provide insight from the experiential director's perspective, as well.

Case Question

TR is getting ready for the annual residency advisory committee retreat. The goal of this meeting is to propose changes in the residency program and also for each preceptor to complete a self-evaluation of his or her precepting skills. What types of preceptor development resources could TR suggest to the committee that could provide on-demand preceptor training and not require the department to invest significant time into developing training materials?

PRECEPTORS-IN-TRAINING

Preceptor-in-training is a term used to describe new preceptors within a pharmacy residency program who are seeking to become qualified preceptors. Such practitioners may be new practitioners or experienced practitioners who are participating in a residency training program for the first time.

ASHP has set forth requirements of preceptors-in-training[2]:

1. They must be assigned an advisor or coach who is a qualified preceptor
2. They must develop a documented preceptor development plan to meet the qualifications for becoming a residency preceptor within 2 years
3. They must not be PGY1 residents

To meet the aforementioned criteria, preceptors-in-training should consider:

♦ Identifying a mentor who has a teaching style that they would like to emulate as a preceptor
♦ Developing a plan of mentoring meetings/discussions related to teaching and learning

---

Case Question

As a preceptor-in-training, TR hopes to identify a mentor who has established new pharmacy services while taking on learners in a similar environment. What are some key qualities of a preceptor TR would look for in a mentor?

To begin the preceptor-in-training process, interested individuals should consider submitting a letter of intent to the residency program director. This letter may include information about you, your practice site, a discussion of reasons why teaching is important or desirable, and how learners may impact your practice and professional development. Along with a letter of intent, consider submitting a teaching philosophy to give the reader an idea of your teaching methods and beliefs.

Additional information and activities related to the initial assessment of the preceptor that should be available include the following[7]:

♦ Description of your qualifications to serve as a preceptor
♦ Interview with residency program director (including a discussion of why you are interested in precepting and your understanding of precepting roles and responsibilities)
♦ Preceptor self-assessment

If you are hoping to precept IPPE or APPE students, consider reaching out to the experiential director at an affiliated college or school of pharmacy to express your interest in precepting learners. Each state may have specific requirements for taking experiential learners, specifications related to precepting criteria, and procedures to obtain a designation as a preceptor.

The path to full preceptor may include completion and review of the following ongoing assessments:

- Resident and student pharmacist evaluations
- Residency program director's, mentor's, or advisor's observations of your precepting
- Preceptor self-assessments
- Peer evaluations

In addition to these assessments, ongoing development should prepare the preceptor-in-training to achieve full preceptor status within a 2-year time frame.[2]

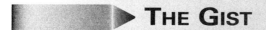 **THE GIST**

1. Self-assessment and preceptor development are deliberative activities that can often fall to the wayside if not made intentionally part of your practice.
2. Developing methods of gathering feedback from both learners and key stakeholders (residency directors, experiential directors, colleagues, etc.) can be helpful in reinforcing or adding to one's self-assessment.
3. Preceptors should continuously seek professional development activities that will advance their skills and knowledge of best practices in precepting.

SUGGESTED READING

ASHP. Articles related to precepting on the ASHP website. http://www.ashp.org/menu/PracticePolicy/ResourceCenters/PreceptorSkills/Articles.aspx

ASHP. Mentoring and preceptor development: paying it forward. http://www.ashp.org/menu/MemberCenter/SectionsForums/NPF/Getting-Started/Mentoring-Preceptor-Development.html

ASHP. ASHP's Section Advisory Group on Preceptor Skills Development. http://www.ashp.org/menu/MemberCenter/SectionsForums/SCSS/AboutThisSection/SAG-on-Preceptor-Skills.aspx

REFERENCES

1. 2015 PGY1 Residency Accreditation Standards Guidance Document Summary of Changes. American Society of Health-System Pharmacists. Available from: http://www.ashp.org/DocLibrary/Accreditation/Regulations-Standards/Summary-of-Guidance-Document-Changes-September-2015.pdf (accessed 27 Nov 2015).
2. ASHP. ASHP Accreditation Standard for Postgraduate Year One (PGY1) Pharmacy Residency Programs. Available from: http://www.ashp.org/DocLibrary/Accreditation/Newly-approved-PGY1-Standard-September-2014.pdf (accessed 28 Feb 2016).

3. ASHP. ASHP Accreditation Standard for Postgraduate Year Two (PGY2) Pharmacy Residency Programs. https://www.ashp.org/DocLibrary/Accreditation/ASD-PGY2-Standard.aspx (accessed 27 Nov 2015).

4. Accreditation Council for Pharmacy Education. Standard 20: Preceptors. In: Accreditation Standards and Key Elements for the Professional Program in Pharmacy Leading to the Doctor of Pharmacy Degree: Standards 2016. 2015. https://www.acpe-accredit.org/pdf/Standards2016FINAL.pdf (accessed 27 Nov 2015).

5. Haase KK, Smythe MA, Orlando PL et al. Quality Experiential Education. *Pharmacotherapy* 2008; 28:219e-27e.

6. ASHP. Preceptor Development and Assessment. 2012. http://www.ashp.org/DocLibrary/Accreditation/Residency-Learning-System/RTP-Preceptor-Assessment-and-Development-Example.aspx (accessed 1 Mar 2016).

7. Ricchetti C, Jun A. Strategies and resources for successful preceptor development. *Am J Health Syst.* 2011; 68:1837-42.

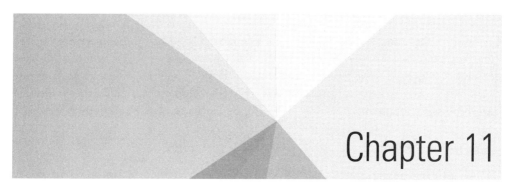

Chapter 11

Using Learners to Improve Your Practice Site

Lukas Everly

CASE STUDY

JR is a new practitioner who had recently taken a position as a generalist within a new healthcare system. Following her residency training, she had a strong desire to precept students and has been a preceptor for the past few years. Although the experiences have been going well, JR would like to develop the rotation to further broaden her students' experience while providing more value to her organization.

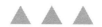

INTRODUCTION

After successfully hosting your first rotation, you may feel like it is time to sit back and admire the fruits of your labor. Once you have a solid learning experience created, however, there is no better time to contemplate the many ways that you can use your learners to improve your practice and expand the experiential offerings at your site. Although giving back to the profession is reason enough to precept learners, the relationship between you and your trainees will be even better if it is mutually beneficial.

LEADING CHANGE

Before you can make any significant changes, you may find it beneficial to review some of the principles of change management. Implementing or supporting a service line with student pharmacists requires a clear vision of your patient population, the skills that students will need to be successful, and what outcomes should be assessed to show results. Any change introduced into an existing system can be met with various challenges either from the learners or other personnel. *Change models* are structured processes that can increase the likelihood that a change is accepted and maintained within an institution. Various models focusing on navigating change are available, but this chapter will focus primarily on models of healthcare or pharmacy services.[1,2] As the profession of pharmacy has progressed through practice model initiatives and focuses on advancement, data regarding the efficacy of change management within pharmacy are available and can serve as a valuable resource in designing new services with the greatest likelihood to last. The Holland-Nimmo Practice Change Model proposes that before any change can be implemented, three characteristics must be satisfied simultaneously: *practice environment, learning resources,* and *motivational strategies.*[4] With respect to practice environment, practitioners are unlikely to adopt a change if they cannot use the new process in their practice. Additionally, receivers of care play a crucial role in shaping the practice environment based on their needs and expectations. With regard to learning resources, they must be useful and easily accessible to allow others to acquire necessary knowledge or skill. Last, the individual must be motivated to take action to institute the change.

One might also consider a change model that is not centered on healthcare. Advantages to this approach include flexibility and ease of integration into your everyday experiences while navigating yourself or others through change. One model with widespread utility would be Prosci's ADKAR (**A**wareness, **D**esire, **K**nowledge, **A**bility, and **R**einforcement) model.[3]

To promote awareness, you should follow a basic framework:

- Orient people to the current situation and rationale for the change.
- Provide details about the change (scope, objectives, time frame, and the amount of change needed).
- Explain how the change impacts the people around you.
- Provide a basic roadmap for the change process (major milestones, overall schedule for the project, and early successes).

Once everyone is aware that a change is necessary, effective leaders must build enthusiasm and interest to ensure that the change process gains momentum. To build interest in the proposed change, there must be a personal context for why the change is beneficial. Before this context can be delivered, change managers must listen and try to understand the viewpoints of those affected by the change. Empathy is a powerful tool to gather information and convey understanding to persons who may be resistant to change. Once this is achieved, managers effect change by removing barriers, creating hope, showing tangible benefits, converting strong dissenters, or by making personal appeals. Although a variety of these tactics may be used, each situation may require a different approach to create a desire for change.

Knowledge refers to the information gained when trying to understand the change, as well as the information on how to change. To effectively use knowledge, it must be readily available, focus on the structure and process of the future state, and clearly convey the skills and behaviors that people will need to operate within the future state. The way that this knowledge is structured and delivered should be dependent on the first two steps of the model to avoid common pitfalls in providing people with information of which they are unaware or have no desire to utilize.

Ability represents the degree to which a person is able to utilize knowledge. Providing awareness, desire, and knowledge is essential to ensuring an environment that nurtures change. The change process often requires people to develop new skills and processes, approach old problems in new ways, or to interact with information or other people differently. From a developmental viewpoint, the ability to change can encompass motor skills, cognitive ability, and even social or behavioral aspects. The same way that precepting learners requires direct instruction, modeling, coaching, and facilitation, effective change agents lead people through the change process.

Finally, *reinforcement* is an important concept to ensure that changes are maintained over time rather than adopted and forgotten as people fall back into old habits. Reinforcement can either be focused on globally promoting and recognizing those who have adopted the change well or by focusing on the specific resistances that arise throughout the process. Overall, ADKAR is useful because of its simplicity and provides a framework on how to approach people through the conceptualization, implementation, and reinforcing stages of implementing meaningful change.

Quick Tip

Many types of change models exist. Find or modify the one that blends best with your own style and environment.

GROWING EXPERIENTIAL OPPORTUNITIES

Establishing your rotation can be the first step on the road to turning your practice site into a flourishing training ground. Although you may have started by hosting a single student or resident, the lessons learned from these first experiences can help you progress to offering rotations for multiple trainees, establishing a pharmacy residency program, or cultivating other staff members into additional preceptors for their own rotations. There are numerous efficiencies that can be identified once you use the recommendations in this text to design or redesign your experiential offerings.

For most practice sites, adding an additional student or resident to an existing rotation can allow you to cover additional services, provide extra manpower to complete projects and will lead to extra opportunities for you to stay abreast of best practices. Look for ways to delegate tasks across a larger number of learners. If possible, you may even consider dispersing your learners across different locations so that you can divide and conquer instead of having a gaggle of trainees trailing behind you each day. Although the addition of an extra learner will increase the time required to complete evaluations and provide feedback, the learners themselves can be used as pharmacist extenders to deliver some of the lectures, assessments, and patient care responsibilities normally provided by the preceptor, freeing up time in the process.

Quick Tip

If you are taking on multiple learners at the same time, using the learners to peer review presentations, journal clubs, or case presentations can allow for a robust assessment of trainee performance without requiring the preceptor to do all of the assessments.

If you have experience precepting students, you may see an opportunity to expand into the realm of resident training. The benefits of establishing a residency program are numerous and have been well documented elsewhere.[4] These trainees are fully functioning pharmacists seeking advanced training. As such, residents can perform high-level tasks that students are not able to complete. For instance, residents can provide direct patient care, verify prescriptions, conduct longitudinal research projects, and serve as preceptors for pharmacy students. Demand for pharmacy residency training has never been higher, and the number of applicants far outpaces the number of available positions each year. On the other hand, establishing a residency can be a daunting endeavor with numerous requirements and standards. ASHP provides resources to help preceptors establish and gain accreditation for pharmacy residency programs.[5] Although the initial investment in program development and accreditation may be significant, the rewards of creating such a program far outweigh any up-front costs.

Another avenue to expand experiential offerings at your site includes other pharmacist coworkers. Chances are that there are a number of pharmacists in your department who have a wealth of knowledge and experience that they can share with trainees. You can serve as a role model and guide to these other practitioners as they consider taking on student and resident rotations. Share your experiences (and the rewards of taking a trainee) with others in your department. Use the knowledge you have gained to help them develop their own learning experience, assessment plan, and teaching skills. When a culture of teaching and learning is established across your department, the benefits will extend to your practice, students, and patients.

> ### *Case Question*
>
> *JR has had great success with her rotations for students. Her service is thriving, and she has made a significant impact on patient care. At the moment, she is one of a small handful of preceptors in her department. Who else could be targeted to expand experiential offerings at her site? How can JR parlay her success with student rotations into the establishment of a pharmacy residency program?*

LEARNERS AS PHARMACIST EXTENDERS

As described above, the benefits of a rotation do not need to flow only in the direction of the learners. Bringing trainees into your practice can dramatically improve your own knowledge, services, and workload. Instead of using learners only in a shadowing role (where their main responsibility is to observe the preceptor as he or she completes his or her duties), place trainees in frontline roles with defined responsibilities so that their efforts can directly impact your patients. Consider advanced roles that students are well prepared to complete. Examples may include patient counseling, attendance on rounds, health screenings, brown bag events, and medication therapy management phone calls. Look for opportunities in your practice that would be easy to implement if you had additional staff to provide the service. Although, ideally, there should be an adequate number of pharmacy personnel to provide them, finding a way to expand or support services without increasing staffing is a more lean approach that many volunteer pharmacy preceptors use.[6] Additional staff will enable you to reach a wider number of patients than would have been possible without the help of your trainees. The increased productivity and impact of your service will more than outweigh the learner training, assessment, and paperwork that follow.

Quick Tip

It is important to note that including students in advanced activities will require an investment in training and orientation. Student and resident competency will vary so you should provide a solid foundation at the start of the rotation so that all trainees can meet your expectations and provide advanced services.

Preceptors using learners to provide advanced services must learn to balance the success of the learner and the service. There are numerous ways to utilize students and residents as pharmacist extenders to address this objective. The main push is to build a structure that allows students to operate semi-independently to provide direct patient care services while also packaging this responsibility in accordance to the type of rotation. For example, learners in an inpatient setting may be asked to provide medication education to the patients who were seen on rounds earlier in the day. If the preceptor were to identify a pressing need for improved pain management or transitions of care, these areas could be the primary targets for learner-led initiatives. Because students and residents would, ideally, be familiar with the target patients, they could serve as a valuable link between patient and provider. If there are misunderstandings or loose ends, the learner can spot them and remedy the situation before any harm is done. In this manner, the learner is improving patient care and helping the institution meet quality improvement metrics. At the same time, the preceptor is responsible for ensuring that the learners are obtaining the experiences and training that will meet the rotation's objectives. It may be enticing to put students to work on a service that is a dire need for the institution, but provides little value to the trainee. This tendency must be resisted so that each party can benefit mutually from the rotation experience. Although learners are an efficient resource in meeting these outcomes, their development needs to remain the primary concern.

Residents, in particular, can fulfill an important role when it comes to expanding pharmacy services. Residents bring a much greater breadth of clinical knowledge, ability, and superior time management skills compared to students. In instances where both residents and students are present, a layered learning model approach is likely the best option. This approach allows students to function with an additional layer of support with the resident serving as a copreceptor. At the same time, the residents develop mentorship skills that they will need in the future when they take over as a primary preceptor.

Case Question

JR learns of a major push from the hospital administration to improve patient satisfaction measures. One medical floor, in particular, is underperforming on metrics of medication education and perception of pain control. How might JR use different learners (students, technicians, interns, or residents) to target medication education and patient satisfaction on the underperforming medical floor?

Quick Tip

Subtle shifts in culture may occur over time when learners are used to grow or sustain new services. Actively surveying the learning environment and seeking feedback from learners ensures that students and residents are not being viewed as free labor.

DEVELOPING THE PRECEPTING SKILLS OF RESIDENTS

Although residents spend a year or longer navigating a residency program, there may be aspects of the program's structure and design that they do not fully understand. An example of this is evident in the residents' self-evaluations. Typical submissions from residents early in the year are essentially lists of the projects and work accomplished during a given rotation, rather than an introspective evaluation of their ability and actionable steps on how to improve. One benefit of imparting preceptor skills to residents is to improve their ability to accurately assess their own development and provide input on how the residency program is functioning. Beyond the future rewards that residents reap from developing preceptor skills, they can also support learners and preceptors in a variety of ways. Preceptors frequently report that work limitations impact the time spent directly with their students and may affect the quality of experiential offerings.[7]

Residents, with appropriate training, can be used as preceptor extenders to:

♦ further support students,
♦ prevent preceptor burn out,
♦ allow preceptors the flexibility to focus on other responsibilities, and
♦ serve as additional resources and sources of feedback for student learners while extending the reach of the department into other areas of the healthcare environment.

Although residents can develop their preceptor skills in a number of ways (continuing education programs, didactic resources, journal articles, or even this text), a more layered approach would allow residents to spend time serving as a copreceptor and self-reflecting on the experience. Once they are more comfortable in the preceptor role, consider assigning them to precept a student of their own. Give your residents the opportunity to develop a syllabus, assessments, and summative evaluations. At each step in the process, serve as a guide to keep the residents on track while still allowing them to be the primary preceptors for the students. Following these recommendations will set your residents up for success and increase the likelihood that they will continue to precept students throughout their careers.

PRECEPTING TECHNICIANS AND INTERNS WITH A DESIRE TO EXPAND ROLES

Beyond students or residents, pharmacy technicians are another group within a pharmacy who can expand services and benefit by exhibiting the roles of a preceptor. Expansion of technician roles and responsibilities has been a supported aspect of practice advancement for a number of years. Technicians who show an innate desire or motivation to try new things or take leadership roles should be quickly identified and supported. With something as simple as a performance improvement project, a technician could be coached through the process of collecting data, analyzing results, and disseminating the results for the benefit of others. Using the available talent by nurturing technicians who are able to function at the height of their abilities can vastly improve the efficiency needed for a pharmacist to provide a high level of service. Developing the technician staff also adds another layer of support for learners at the rotation site. Technicians engaged within a service, who are well versed in the day-to-day operations, are equipped to handle many procedural or structural questions and can facilitate a smooth orientation for learners navigating a new environment. Similarly, pharmacy interns mirror many qualities of advanced technicians, especially early in their training. A key difference is the speed at which they progress, in part due to their ongoing academic development. Interns also represent an often underutilized group that may be actively seeking additional roles and responsibilities.

LEARNERS AS INNOVATORS AND CATALYSTS

An additional benefit to precepting is the ability to use students and residents to impact the culture and scope of your pharmacy department. Trainees generally are a motivated, energetic group, eager to make an impact on patients and the department. If you are considering implementing a new service, seriously contemplate how you can incorporate learners into the new process. Residents are required to complete a project over the course of their training, and a number of learning objectives cover the skills that are required to develop, implement, and assess new services.

Your trainees can become a small army to help you collect outcomes data as a source of scholarship and help you disseminate your findings to other practitioners across your institution or across the country. In an ideal setting, a layered model could be used with a primary preceptor supporting a resident who then uses students for aspects of conducting a research project. Faculty often employ a similar approach to build a sustainable "scholarship engine."[8] The student may be assigned to more superficial responsibilities, such as data collection. Although this may serve the overall direction of the project, it is important to ensure that any student assisting with research gains a functional understanding on how to conduct research. Sharing information on why particular outcomes were chosen, the types of conclusions the results may show, and what statistical analysis will be used are all examples of balancing student value versus development. In the case of learners seeking to develop their own original research projects, Table 11-1 can be used as a guide to help build a specific and measurable research question.

Because students generally spend less time onsite, expecting them to enact meaningful change is often a lofty goal. For residents, however, it is very feasible to see meaningful contributions to the practice site each year. As described above, residents are required to complete a major project over the course of the year and a number of specific goals and objectives assess their abilities to do so. In addition to their use in performance improvement projects, a core piece of any residency program is a staffing component. This responsibility to practice as a pharmacist is meant to build skills in clinical judgment and independence. Participating as staff members, residents spend additional time onsite working with more types of practitioners, such as nurses, physicians, administration, and other departments as they fill different roles within the department. Thanks to these far-reaching connections, they can serve a crucial role as change agents. Residents may find themselves in a strange middle ground, privy to information from management and unfiltered opinion from within the department. As change agents, residents have a favorable combination of expertise, minimal direct authority, and potentially the greatest familiarity with other members of the department. Using this unique combination allows them to provide feedback to department leadership, support communication among the staff, provide training to the staff regarding a new process or service, and identify pockets of support or resistance to new initiatives. Some residents may even find themselves piloting new services as a component of their research project for the year. A resident project that evaluates the outcomes, feasibilities, and cost implications of a new service line can be directly translatable to process improvement within the department.

Learners fulfill a multitude of roles within various practice settings and should exhibit the skills and knowledge they develop during an experience. By carefully researching, structuring, integrating, and supporting the experiential rotation, preceptors ensure that they are providing high-quality learning experiences for trainees that also improve patient outcomes.

Table 11-1. Developing a Research Question and Study Design

Step 1: Develop a one-sentence research question using the FINER criteria[a]

F—Feasible. Is the question answerable? Do you have access to all the materials you will need to do the study? Do you have access to enough subjects? Will you have enough time and money? Do you have the expertise or access to a collaborator?

I—Interesting. Is the research interesting to the investigator and targeted population?

N—Novel. Has this study been done before? How does it add to the current knowledge base?

E—Ethical. Can the study be done in a way that does not subject patients to excess risks? Will an institutional review board approve the study?

R—Relevant. Will it further medical science? Will the results change practice or focus?

Step 2: Develop specific aims and/or a hypothesis

In one sentence, express your specific aims or hypothesis of the project. It should be well defined, important, and feasible

Step 3: Set forth background and significance

Why is your research question important? Perform a search of the current literature pertaining to your research question. Describe the existing evidence (including citations) and how your project will contribute. Identify any gaps in existing knowledge that can be addressed by your research. Stress any innovations in your experimental design.

Suggested structure:
* Rationale for the proposed project
* State of existing knowledge (literature review)
* Identify gaps that your project intends to fill
* Cite your sources within your rationale

Step 4: Describe your study's design and methods

Describe the following components of your study:
* Study design (cohort study, retrospective chart review, clinical trial, etc.)
* Primary outcome and data type (continuous, nominal, ordinal)
* Study population (inclusion/exclusion criteria)

Study design:

Primary outcome:

Inclusion:

Exclusion:

[a]See Reference 9 for more information about FINER criteria.

Case Question

JR has identified a situation in which learners could be used to improve care. She has decided to have pharmacy students reside on medical floors to serve as a resource for nursing, provide patient education, round with the medical team, and conduct patient interviews for patients reporting pain scores greater than 5 out of 10. What qualities will students need to be successful? How can JR work with the other care providers to be a change leader and facilitate this additional student involvement to ensure its success?

THE GIST

1. Assess the current needs of your practice site to ensure student services are targeting meaningful outcomes.
2. While pharmacist extenders (students, interns, technicians) are a cost-effective way to grow services, their growth and development must be a key focus.
3. A layered learning model with residents and students providing services requires close attention to the development of precepting skills and independence of each group to ensure smooth operation.
4. Learners can serve an additional role as change agents within a department via performance improvement projects, research studies, formulary activities, and staff training.

SUGGESTED READING

Nguyen KA, Hart SR, Pidcock KN et al. Creating learning opportunities for pharmacy students through an observation program. *Am J Health-Syst Pharm.* 2012; 69:1905-9.

Rathbun RC, Hester EK, Arnold LM. Importance of patient care in advanced pharmacy practice experiences. *Pharmacotherapy.* 2012; 65:285-92.

Williams MF, Towne TG, Griffin SE. Developing a practice site in the nonacademic community hospital: a primer for pharmacy practice faculty members. *Curr Pharm Teach Learn.* 2015; 7:899-907.

REFERENCES

1. Holland RW, Nimmo CM. Transitions in pharmacy practice, part 3: effecting change—the three-ring circus. *Am J Health-Syst Pharm.* 1999; 56:2235-41.
2. Harris IM, Baker E, Berry TM et al. Developing a business-practice model for pharmacy services in ambulatory settings. *Pharmacotherapy.* 2008; 28:285.

3. Hiatt JM. ADKAR: a model for change in business, government and our community. *How to Implement Successful Change in Our Personal Lives and Professional Careers.* London: Prosci Research; 1998.

4. Smith KM, Sorensen T, Connor KA et al. Value of conducting pharmacy residency training—the organization perspective. *Pharmacotherapy.* 2010; 30:490e-510e.

5. Ross SR, Swanson K, Bot JA. How to start a residency program: what you really need to know. Nelson BA, ed. ASHP Accreditation Services Division, 2015. https://www.ashp.org/DocLibrary/Accreditation/Starting-Residency/RTP-HowStartResidencyPrgm.aspx (accessed 29 Apr 2016).

6. Delgado O, Kernan WP, Knoer SJ. Advancing the pharmacy practice model in a community teaching hospital by expanding student rotations. *Am J Health-Syst Pharm.* 2014; 17:1871-6.

7. Skrabal MZ, Jones RM, Nemire RE et al. National survey of volunteer pharmacy preceptors. *Am J Pharm Educ.* 2008; 72(5):112.

8. Galal SM, Carr-Lopez SM, Gomez S et al. A collaborative approach to combining service, teaching, and research. *Am J Pharm Educ.* 2014; 78(3):58.

9. Hulley SB, Cummings SR, Browner WS et al. *Designing Clinical Research.* 3rd ed. Philadelphia: Lippincott Williams & Wilkins; 2007.

Index

A

Action, 76–77
Activities
    calendar/day-planner for, 9
    prioritization of, 9
ADKAR (awareness, desire, knowledge, ability and reinforcement) model, 148–149
Advanced pharmacy practice experiences (APPEs), 18–20, 27
    evaluation of, 113–117
ASHP
    accreditation standards, 20
    preceptor self-assessment, 143
Assessment
    feedback vs. 70
    of IPPEs, 17
    of practice site, 3–6
    of preceptor, 135–141
Attendance policy, 32

B

Baseline testing, 51
Behaviors, student, 48
Boyle, Jaclyn, 135–146

C

Cardiologist, 5
Cardiology rotation, 47
Career development, 125
    mission statement, 126, 127–128
    values in, 125–126
Case presentation(s), 33–34
    evaluation of, 83–84
Case-based teaching, 60
Change management, 148
Change models, 148
Chart review, 63
Coaching, 59, 77

Cognitive learning, 57
Come out with bad news, 76
Communication issues, 95–97
Communication skills, 64–65
    assessing, 65
Community-based APPEs, 19
Community-based IPPEs, 15
Competency
    patient care, 40–41
    teaching, education and knowledge dissemination, 41–42
Corrective feedback, 74
Critical thinking
    activities, 67
    teaching, 61–63
Curriculum vitae review, 50

D

Debriefing, 63
Deductive reasoning, 62
Dietitian, 5
Difficult situations, 87–88
Direct instruction, 57–59
Direct observation, 51
Disinterested learners, 93–94

E

Emotional intelligence, 63–66, 88
    activities, 67
    assessing, 66–67
    competencies, 64
Emotional learner, 99–100
English as second language students, 95–96
Entitled learners, 92–93
Errors, handling, 100–101
e-Technology, 89
Evaluation
    APPE, 113–117
    case presentation, 83–84
    journal club, 81–82

Everly, Lukas, 147–157
Exit interviews, 137–138

F

Facilitation, 59–60
Fast learners, 97, 101–102
Feedback, 69, 70–72
    approaches to, 73–76
    assessment vs. 70–71
    of colleagues, superiors, 142
    effective, 72, 80
    giving difficult, 76–78
    key principles of, 72–73
    learner and, 136
    sandwich, 73, 95
Final evaluation, 33, 106–112
    feedback and, 108
    poor performance presentation in, 110
    presentation of, 109–110
Five Minute Preceptor teaching model, 60–61
Formative assessment, 70

G

Goal setting, preceptor, 141
Goals, 125
Grade inflation, 108

H

Healthcare professional interactions, 16
Honors grade, 111
Hospital outpatient pharmacy site assessment, 3–6

I

Inductive reasoning, 62
Informal feedback, 136
Institution-based APPEs, 19
Institution-based IPPEs, 15
Interns, precepting, 153

Introductory pharmacy practice experiences (IPPEs), 13, 14–17, 27
    patient care activities for, 15

L

Laboratory manager, 5
Layered-learning model (LLM), 14, 24–26, 27
    challenges, 25–26
Learner(s)
    baseline testing of, 51
    direct observation of, 51
    discussions with, 50
    disinterested, 93–94
    emotional, 99–100
    entitled, 92–93
    fast, 97, 101–103
    feedback and, 136
    getting to know, 49–52
    as innovators and catalysts, 154
    overconfident, 94–95
    previous evaluations of, 50
    as pharmacist extenders, 151–152
    progression expectations for, 34
    struggling, 101–103
    unprepared, 91–92
Learning experience
    activities and goals/objectives evaluation of, 40–42
    calendar for, 44
    description of, 29–30
    evaluation strategy for, 43
    expected progression of resident responsibilities in, 42
    purpose of, 30–31
    sample of, 37–39
Learning material, customization, 53
Learning objective grid, 7–8
Learning styles, 102
Lecture capture products, 53

Letters of recommendation, 129–130, 131, 134
Listening, 77
Logistics, 49

M

Medication therapy management (MTM) services, 6
Mentor, 88
    effective, 123–124
Mentoring, 122–123
    moments, 125
    phases of, 123, 124
    solution-focused, 123, 124
Midpoint evaluation, 78–79, 107
Mission statement, 126, 127–128
Modeling, 49, 59, 96

N

Networking, 130, 132–133
    activities, 134
Next steps, 22

O

Orientation, 25, 47, 54
    customizing, 52
    modeling session for, 49
    syllabus review and expectations for, 48
    time savers in, 53–54
Overconfident learners, 94–95

P

Patient
    care activities, IPPEs, 14–15
    case problem list, 7
    -related outcomes, 24
Patient counseling, 16, 52, 53
    rubric, 85–86
Patient safety officer, 5
Pendleton Four-Step Model, 74
Personality issues, biases, 98
Pharmacy technician, 5

Physical therapist, 5
Portfolio review, 50
Post evaluation, 79
Postcompletion surveys, 138
Postgraduate year 1 residency (PGY1), 20–22, 27
Postgraduate year 2 residency (PGY2), 23, 27
Practice, 156
    experiential opportunities in, 149–150
    strengths, determining, 4–5
Practice improvement, 147–148
    change and, 148
    learners as innovators and catalysts in, 154
    learners as pharmacist extenders in, 151
    precepting technicians, interns to expand roles in, 153
    research question, study design development for, 155
Praise, 77
Preceptor
    contact, 31
    evaluation/assessment, 11, 135–141, 143
    interaction, 10
    learner feedback to, 136–137
    roles of, 57–60
    self-assessment by, 138–139, 141, 143
Preceptor development, 135, 141–143
    plan, 141
    resources, 142
Preceptors-in-training, 144–145
Prioritization, 90
Procrastination, 91
Professional development, preceptor, 141–142
Professionalism, 16, 88–90, 103

R

Reflection, 66

Reframing bad news, 76

Reinforcing feedback, 73, 74

Research question development, 155

Resident
   development of precepting skills, 152–153
   training, 150–152

Rotation
   activities scheduling in, 9–10
   classification of, 9
   contingency projects for, 10
   curriculum of topics for, 10
   customizing, 52–53
   day-to-day activities development in, 9–10
   goals and objectives framework for, 6–7
   ongoing formative feedback during, 107
   selection of, 4
   staggering start times for, 54
   tailoring, 13
   trainee file for, 52
   training and logistics in, 49
   unmatched activities and, 9
   wrapping up, 105–6

S

Schneider, Stacey R., 55–68, 87–104, 121–134

Self-assessment/ self-evaluation, 60, 110, 125

preceptor, 138–138

Self-efficacy, 124

Simulated scenarios, 63

Site assessment, 3–4
   practice strengths, 4–5
   practice weaknesses, 5–6

Situation-Behavior-Impact (SBI) Feedback Tool, 73–75

Skilled nursing facility nurse, 5

SMART goals, 91, 139

Social media, 133

Social worker, 5

Solution-focused mentoring, 123, 124

Soric, Mate M., 3–12, 29–44, 47–54

Specificity, 76

StrengthsFinder 2.0, 123

Struggling learners, 101

Study design development, 155

Summative assessment, 70
   preceptor evaluations, 136–137

Supplemental preceptors, 5

SWOT (strengths, weaknesses, opportunities, threats) analysis, 139, 140

Syllabus
   assessment plan, assignments in, 33–34
   attendance policy in, 32
   calendar in, 33
   delivery to learners, 34–35
   general description and logistics in, 31–32
   goals, objectives, activities

and, 32–33
   learner progression expectations in, 34
   off-hours activities and, 32
   preceptor contact and, 31
   purpose of, 30, 31, 35
      review and expectations of, 48
   writing, 29–30

T

Task completion, 22

Taxonomy of Educational Objectives, 7

Teaching
   critical thinking skills, 61–63
   emotional intelligence, 63
   other strategies, 62–63
   Socratic method of, 62

Teaching philosophy, 55
   sample, 58
   writing, 56–57

Technicians, precepting and, 153

Thinking aloud, 62

Time management, 21, 90, 92

Training, 49

Transition of care, layered-learning model, 25

U, V, W

Undergrading, 109

Unprepared learners, 91–92

Values, 125–126

Wisneski, S. Scott, 13–28, 69–86, 105–117

Work–personal life balance, 91

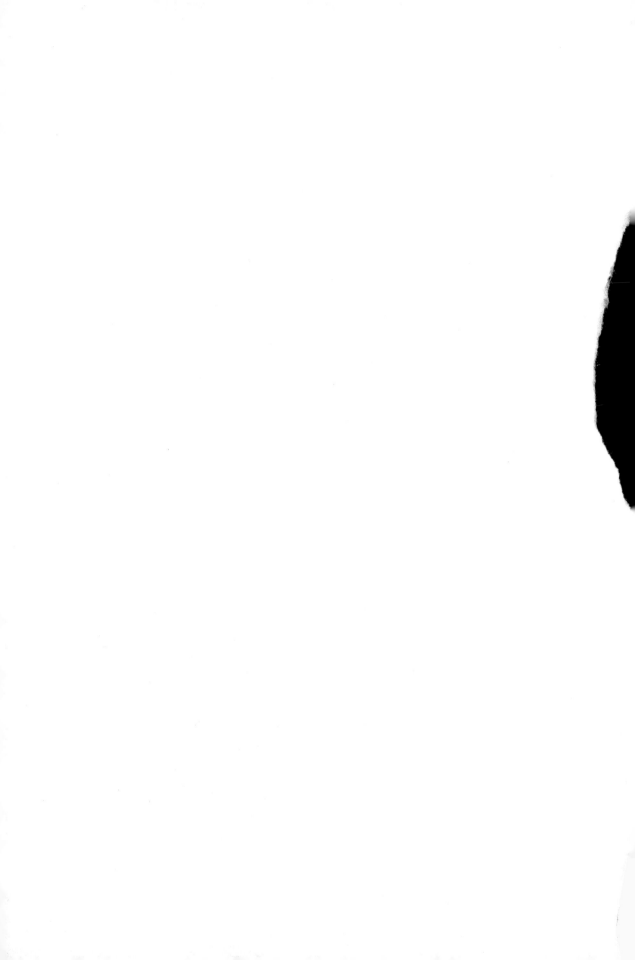